Preparedness, Response, and Recovery Considerations for Children and Families

Workshop Summary

Theresa Wizemann, Megan Reeve, and Bruce M. Altevogt,
Rapporteurs

Forum on Medical and Public Health Preparedness for Catastrophic Events

Board on Health Sciences Policy

INSTITUTE OF MEDICINE
OF THE NATIONAL ACADEMIES

THE NATIONAL ACADEMIES PRESS
Washington, D.C.
www.nap.edu

THE NATIONAL ACADEMIES PRESS • 500 Fifth Street, NW • Washington, DC 20001

NOTICE: The workshop that is the subject of this workshop summary was approved by the Governing Board of the National Research Council, whose members are drawn from the councils of the National Academy of Sciences, the National Academy of Engineering, and the Institute of Medicine.

This activity was supported by contracts between the National Academy of Sciences and the American College of Emergency Physicians; American Hospital Association; Association of State and Territorial Health Officials; Centers for Disease Control and Prevention (Contract No. 200-2011-38807, TO #19); Department of Defense (Contract No. HT0011-11-P-0186); Department of Defense, Uniformed Services University of the Health Sciences (Contract No. HT9404-12-1-0022); Department of Health and Human Services' National Institutes of Health: National Institute of Allergy and Infectious Diseases, National Institute of Environmental Sciences, National Library of Medicine (Contract No. HHSN26300007 [Under Base 1 #HHSN263201200074I]); Department of Health and Human Services' Office of the Assistant Secretary for Preparedness and Response (Contract No. HHSO100201000021P); Department of Homeland Security's Federal Emergency Management Agency (Contract No. HSFE20-13-P-0212); Department of Homeland Security, Office of Health Affairs (Contract No. HSHQDC-13-J-00384 [Under Base 1 #HSHQDC-11-D-00009]); Department of Transportation's National Highway Traffic Safety Administration (Contract No. DTNH22-10-H-00287); Department of Veterans Affairs (Contract No. 101-G09041); Emergency Nurses Association; Food and Drug Administration (Contract No. HHSF22301027T [Under Base Contract DHHS-8598]); Infectious Diseases Society of America; Martin, Blanck & Associates; Mayo Clinic; Merck Research Laboratories (Contract No. 2391); National Association of Chain Drug Stores; National Association of County and City Health Officials; National Association of Emergency Medical Technicians; Pharmaceutical Research and Manufacturers of America; Target Corporation; Trauma Center Association of America; and United Health Foundation. The views presented in this publication do not necessarily reflect the views of the organizations or agencies that provided support for the activity.

International Standard Book Number-13: 978-0-309-29458-4
International Standard Book Number-10: 0-309-29458-4

Additional copies of this workshop summary are available for sale from the National Academies Press, 500 Fifth Street, NW, Keck 360, Washington, DC 20001; (800) 624-6242 or (202) 334-3313; http://www.nap.edu.

For more information about the Institute of Medicine, visit the IOM home page at: **www.iom.edu.**

Printed in the United States of America

Suggested citation: IOM (Institute of Medicine). 2014. *Preparedness, response, and recovery considerations for children and families: Workshop summary.* Washington, DC: The National Academies Press.

"Knowing is not enough; we must apply.
Willing is not enough; we must do."
—Goethe

INSTITUTE OF MEDICINE
OF THE NATIONAL ACADEMIES

Advising the Nation. Improving Health.

THE NATIONAL ACADEMIES

Advisers to the Nation on Science, Engineering, and Medicine

The **National Academy of Sciences** is a private, nonprofit, self-perpetuating society of distinguished scholars engaged in scientific and engineering research, dedicated to the furtherance of science and technology and to their use for the general welfare. Upon the authority of the charter granted to it by the Congress in 1863, the Academy has a mandate that requires it to advise the federal government on scientific and technical matters. Dr. Ralph J. Cicerone is president of the National Academy of Sciences.

The **National Academy of Engineering** was established in 1964, under the charter of the National Academy of Sciences, as a parallel organization of outstanding engineers. It is autonomous in its administration and in the selection of its members, sharing with the National Academy of Sciences the responsibility for advising the federal government. The National Academy of Engineering also sponsors engineering programs aimed at meeting national needs, encourages education and research, and recognizes the superior achievements of engineers. Dr. C. D. Mote, Jr., is president of the National Academy of Engineering.

The **Institute of Medicine** was established in 1970 by the National Academy of Sciences to secure the services of eminent members of appropriate professions in the examination of policy matters pertaining to the health of the public. The Institute acts under the responsibility given to the National Academy of Sciences by its congressional charter to be an adviser to the federal government and, upon its own initiative, to identify issues of medical care, research, and education. Dr. Harvey V. Fineberg is president of the Institute of Medicine.

The **National Research Council** was organized by the National Academy of Sciences in 1916 to associate the broad community of science and technology with the Academy's purposes of furthering knowledge and advising the federal government. Functioning in accordance with general policies determined by the Academy, the Council has become the principal operating agency of both the National Academy of Sciences and the National Academy of Engineering in providing services to the government, the public, and the scientific and engineering communities. The Council is administered jointly by both Academies and the Institute of Medicine. Dr. Ralph J. Cicerone and Dr. C. D. Mote, Jr., are chair and vice chair, respectively, of the National Research Council.

www.national-academies.org

WORKSHOP PLANNING COMMITTEE[1]

MICHAEL ANDERSON (*Chair*), University Hospitals Case Medical Center and Rainbow Babies and Children's Hospital, Cleveland, OH
TERRY ADIRIM, Office of Special Health Affairs, Health Resources and Services Administration, U.S. Department of Health and Human Services, Rockville, MD
WYNDOLYN BELL, UnitedHealthcare, Atlanta, GA
BRUCE CLEMENTS, Community Preparedness Section, Texas Department of State Health Services, Austin
DANIEL DODGEN, Office for At Risk Individuals, Behavioral Health, and Human Services Coordination, Office of the Assistant Secretary for Preparedness and Response, U.S. Department of Health and Human Services, Washington, DC
PATRICIA FROST, Emergency Medical Services, Contra Costa County Health Services, Contra Costa, CA
ANDREW GARRETT, National Disaster Medical System, Office of the Assistant Secretary for Preparedness and Response, U.S. Department of Health and Human Services, Washington, DC
ANN MASTEN, Institute of Child Development, University of Minnesota, Minneapolis
SCOTT NEEDLE, Healthcare Network of Southwest Florida, Naples
GEORGINA PEACOCK, National Center on Birth Defects and Developmental Disabilities, Centers for Disease Control and Prevention, Atlanta, GA
MARY RILEY, Office of Human Services Emergency Preparedness and Response, Administration for Children and Families, U.S. Department of Health and Human Services, Washington, DC
ANDREW RUCKS, Department of Healthcare Organization and Policy, University of Alabama at Birmingham School of Public Health
KENNETH W. SCHOR, National Center for Disaster Medicine and Public Health, Uniformed Services University of the Health Sciences, Bethesda, MD
CHRISTINE TUCK, National Association of School Nurses, Topeka, KS

---

[1]Institute of Medicine planning committees are solely responsible for organizing the workshop, identifying topics, and choosing speakers. The responsibility for the published workshop summary rests with the workshop rapporteurs and the institution.

IOM Staff

BRUCE M. ALTEVOGT, Project Director
MEGAN REEVE, Associate Program Officer
KATE KELLEY, Research Associate (*through August 2013*)
BRADLEY ECKERT, Research Associate (*from October 2013*)
ALEX REPACE, Senior Program Assistant

FORUM ON MEDICAL AND PUBLIC HEALTH PREPAREDNESS FOR CATASTROPHIC EVENTS[1]

---

[1]Institute of Medicine forums and roundtables do not issue, review, or approve individual documents. The responsibility for the published workshop summary rests with the workshop rapporteurs and the institution.

JAMES J. JAMES, Disaster Medicine and Public Health Preparedness, Onancock, VA (*until September 2013*)
PAUL E. JARRIS, Association of State and Territorial Health Officials, Arlington, VA
BRIAN KAMOIE, The White House, Washington, DC (*until September 2013*)
LISA G. KAPLOWITZ, Office of the Assistant Secretary for Preparedness and Response, U.S. Department of Health and Human Services, Washington, DC
ALI S. KHAN, Centers for Disease Control and Prevention, Atlanta, GA
MICHAEL G. KURILLA, National Institute of Allergy and Infectious Diseases, Washington, DC
JAYNE LUX, National Business Group on Health, Washington, DC
LINDA M. MACINTYRE, American Red Cross, San Rafael, CA (*from September 2013*)
SUZET M. MCKINNEY, Chicago Department of Public Health, IL
NICOLE MCKOIN, Target Corporation, Furlong, PA
MARGARET M. MCMAHON, Emergency Nurses Association, Williamstown, NJ
AUBREY K. MILLER, National Institute of Environmental Health Sciences, Bethesda, MD
MATTHEW MINSON, Texas A&M University, College Station
ERIN MULLEN, Pharmaceutical Research and Manufacturers of America, Washington, DC
JOHN OSBORN, Mayo Clinic, Rochester, MN
ANDREW T. PAVIA, Infectious Disease Society of America, Salt Lake City, UT
STEVEN J. PHILLIPS, National Library of Medicine, Bethesda, MD
LEWIS J. RADONOVICH, Department of Veterans Affairs, Washington, DC
KENNETH W. SCHOR, Uniformed Services University of the Health Sciences, Bethesda, MD (*from November 2012*)
ROSLYNE SCHULMAN, American Hospital Association, Washington, DC
RICHARD SERINO, Federal Emergency Management Agency, Department of Homeland Security, Washington, DC
SHARON A. R. STANLEY, American Red Cross, Circleville, OH (*until September 2013*)
ERIC S. TONER, UPMC Center for Health Security, Baltimore, MD (*until September 2013*)

REED V. TUCKSON, UnitedHealth Group, Minnetonka, MN (*until September 2013*)
MARGARET VANAMRINGE, The Joint Commission, Washington, DC
W. CRAIG VANDERWAGEN, Martin, Blanck & Associates, Alexandria, VA (*from February 2013*)
JENNIFER WARD, Trauma Center Association of America, Las Cruces, NM (*from February 2013*)
JOHN M. WIESMAN, Washington State Department of Health, Tumwater (*from September 2013*)
GAMUNU WIJETUNGE, National Highway Traffic Safety Administration, Washington, DC

IOM Staff

BRUCE M. ALTEVOGT, Forum Director
MEGAN REEVE, Associate Program Officer
KATE KELLEY, Research Associate (*until August 2013*)
BRADLEY ECKERT, Research Associate (*from October 2013*)
ALEX REPACE, Senior Program Assistant
ANDREW M. POPE, Director, Board on Health Sciences Policy

Reviewers

This workshop summary has been reviewed in draft form by individuals chosen for their diverse perspectives and technical expertise, in accordance with procedures approved by the National Research Council's Report Review Committee. The purpose of this independent review is to provide candid and critical comments that will assist the institution in making its published workshop summary as sound as possible and to ensure that the workshop summary meets institutional standards for objectivity, evidence, and responsiveness to the study charge. The review comments and draft manuscript remain confidential to protect the integrity of the process. We wish to thank the following individuals for their review of this workshop summary:

ARTHUR COOPER, Harlem Hospital Center
MARY HILFIKER, University of California, San Diego
TALA HOOBAN, U.S. Department of Health and Human Services
ROBERT KANTER, SUNY Upstate Medical University
ANDREW C. RUCKS, University of Alabama at Birmingham

Although the reviewers listed above have provided many constructive comments and suggestions, they did not see the final draft of the workshop summary before its release. The review of this workshop summary was overseen by **KRISTINE GEBBIE,** Flinders University School of Nursing and Midwifery. Appointed by the Institute of Medicine, she was responsible for making certain that an independent examination of this workshop summary was carried out in accordance with institutional procedures and that all review comments were carefully considered. Responsibility for the final content of this workshop summary rests entirely with the rapporteurs and the institution.

Contents

1

Introduction and Overview[1]

Communities across the United States face the threat of emergencies and disasters almost every day, natural and man-made, urban and rural, large and small. Although children represent nearly 25 percent of the U.S. population, current state and local disaster preparedness plans often do not include specific considerations for children and families. The preparedness and resilience of communities related to children will require a systems framework for disaster preparedness across traditional and nontraditional medical and public health stakeholders, including community organizations, schools, and other partners in municipal planning.

BACKGROUND

On June 11 and 12, 2013, the Institute of Medicine Forum on Medical and Public Health Preparedness for Catastrophic Events convened a workshop in Washington, DC, to discuss disaster preparedness, response, and resilience relative to the needs of children and families, including children with special health care needs. Participants included traditional and nontraditional medical and public health stakeholders from across federal, state, and local government,

[1]This report has been prepared by the workshop rapporteurs as a factual summary of what occurred at the workshop. The planning committee's role was limited to planning and convening the workshop. The views contained in the report are those of individual workshop participants and do not necessarily represent the views of all workshop participants, the planning committee, or the Institute of Medicine.

health care coalitions, community organizations, school districts, child care providers, hospitals, private health care providers, insurers, academia, and other partners in municipal planning.

The workshop was designed to review existing tools and frameworks that can be modified to include children's needs; identify child-serving partners and organizations that can be leveraged in planning to improve outcomes for children; highlight best practices in resilience and recovery strategies for children; and raise awareness of the need to integrate children's considerations throughout local and state emergency plans. The specific workshop objectives can be found in Box 1-1.[2]

BOX 1-1
Workshop Objectives

- Discuss progress being made in different sectors around the country related to the 2010 recommendations of the National Commission on Children and Disasters (NCCD; the Commission), and opportunities for integrating related children's disaster preparedness efforts into local and state planning efforts.
- Discuss opportunities to augment children's benefits by leveraging existing coalitions.
    - Explore coalition challenges and successes from federal, state, local, and provider perspectives.
- Describe opportunities to strengthen public health partnerships to address the needs of children and families.
- Understand barriers and challenges to better financial systems related to preparedness for children and families.
    - Discuss importance of health care financing education among stakeholders.
    - Consider strategies to reduce the financial burden on public health and health care facilities.
- Emphasize different capabilities needed for mass care and sheltering to provide for families and children with special health care needs.
- Examine resilience strategies that lead to successful recovery in children after a disaster.
- Understand current approaches and interventions to improve recovery in children after any type of emergency or disaster.

---

[2]A full statement of task can be found in Appendix C.

ABOUT THIS SUMMARY

The report that follows summarizes the presentations and discussions by the expert panelists and participants during the workshop. Chapter 2 provides background on some of the issues surrounding planning for children in disasters, an overview of the recommendations from the 2010 National Commission on Children and Disasters (NCCD) report, and progress thus far in integrating the needs of children into preparedness planning. Chapter 3 discusses leveraging health care coalitions to meet the needs of children in disasters, while Chapter 4 focuses on tools and studies done to augment state and local planning for children. Chapter 5 includes provider, hospital, insurer, and health system perspectives on the challenges of funding preparedness and response activities. The importance of public health partnerships and collaboration with community organizations in planning is discussed in Chapter 6. In Chapter 7, some of the specific needs of children during response are discussed (functional needs, nutritional needs, family reunification, temporary child care). Chapters 8 and 9 focus on the importance of tracking mental and behavioral health recovery of children and families, as well as strategies to foster resilience, and interventions that promote the social and economic well-being of children. Finally, Chapter 10 looks at the recovery experience after Hurricane Sandy from child and family agencies and their plans moving forward. Resources and other materials from the workshop can be found in the appendixes, and, specifically, a paper that was commissioned for this workshop is provided in Appendix G, and a resource list of all the tools mentioned throughout the report can be found in Appendix F.

HIGHLIGHTED TOPICS[3]

Throughout the 2-day workshop, a variety of themes emerged across multiple workshop presentations and discussions. The following topics were highlighted by Anderson and the session chairs in summary statements at the close of the workshop. Each of these topics will be discussed at greater length throughout the report.

---

[3]Rapporteurs' summary based on the presentations, discussions, and summary remarks by the meeting and session chairs.

- **Ongoing concerns:** National advocates remain concerned regarding children's needs and trends. The ability to make progress is impeded by the federal fiscal crisis and competing institutional and organizational priorities. Although the NCCD report provides good baseline recommendations, there are still other areas that need attention.
- **Federal engagement:** Federal partners are engaged and trying to move issues and policies related to children's disaster preparedness forward. There are working groups at the White House, the Department of Health and Human Services, the Federal Emergency Management Agency (FEMA), the Centers for Disease Control and Prevention, and others, and there are actions being taken on the NCCD recommendations.
- **Need for central coordination:** The 2013 Pandemic and All-Hazards Preparedness Act reauthorization includes a new advisory committee on children and disasters, but as of yet it has not been appointed.
- **Lack of centralized information and resources:** Many participants stressed the need for a national clearinghouse of tools and resources. There were numerous examples of tools and trainings shared at the workshop, and many lessons learned and best practices were shared from recent events such as Hurricane Sandy, the tornadoes in Joplin, Missouri, and Moore, Oklahoma, and the Newtown, Connecticut, school shooting. However, there is no centralized location to share these resources across jurisdictions, or any way for those who need them to easily find them. Similarly, there is no central coordination of the various recovery assets available to individuals from federal, state, and local agencies, nonprofit organizations, and others. Since the workshop, the Administration for Children and Families has created a webpage of early childhood disaster resources organized for providers, children and families, and policy makers.[4]
- **Building and sustaining health care coalitions:** Successful coalition building involves sharing information, working together to set and achieve goals, and developing formal relationships of commitment. Throughout the workshop, there

---

[4]See http://www.acf.hhs.gov/programs/ohsepr/early-childhood (accessed November 12, 2013).

were what Anderson called "world-class examples of coalitions." The operational question is how to replicate these examples, and to expand them beyond pediatric providers and hospitals.

- **Broader engagement of stakeholders:** There are many different settings and systems that serve children. Many speakers and participants stressed the need to build partnerships across sectors (e.g., behavioral health, public health, medical services, human services, educational systems, emergency management systems, community organizations) with a constant focus on children as they are, and in the environments where they live. Some participants who had previously worked with only clinical and emergency partners highlighted the need for more training and planning with community partners, and suggested thinking more broadly about collaborating with other child-serving community groups that can contribute to community preparedness.
    - **Youth:** Youth involvement in preparedness fosters resilience, and youth can serve as messengers to their peers and parents. Hearing from Ashley Houston from FEMA's Youth Preparedness Council, it became more apparent that engaging youth today will ensure future generations of better prepared adults. Social media can be a powerful outreach tool.
    - **People with disabilities:** Several presentations stressed the importance of planning for the evacuation, transport, and sheltering needs of children with disabilities or access and functional needs. Presenters said that people with disabilities, or their representatives, should be included in planning groups, and children with disabilities should have a say in their own evacuation and transportation plans when they are old enough.
    - **Community providers/private physicians:** Concerns were raised about the need to better integrate private-sector practitioners into local disaster planning. A key barrier to preparedness at the practice level is the lack of payment for time spent in preparedness activities (as these are not reimbursable).
    - **Child care providers:** Participants at the state and national level raised many child care–related issues, from the importance of getting child care up and running after a

disaster, to temporary child care in shelters, to the difficulties locating and communicating with impacted providers in a disaster, including both family- and center-based providers. Several participants discussed the importance of including child care providers as stakeholders in preparedness planning, and increasing the focus on plans for sheltering in place and communication with parents. They also highlighted barriers to the preparedness, response, and recovery of child care facilities.

- **Financing:** There was much interest in finding new models of financing preparedness efforts and care during disasters to make sure that resilience, preparedness, and response for children and families are integral parts of preparedness planning. As Scott Needle of the Healthcare Network of Southwest Florida highlighted, making the business case for financing preparedness is challenging, as disasters are low-frequency events with a low financial return on investment, but can have a huge economic impact. Insurance reimbursement pays for intervention, not for preparedness. However, hospitals that are more prepared before a disaster will have better outcomes and less need for reimbursement assistance. Participants discussed the relevance of dual use capabilities to preparedness, noting that improved day-to-day operations can reap benefits for emergency preparedness.
- **Ability to surge:** There were many concerns expressed about pediatric bed capacity and the ability to surge when needed, especially noted by Patricia Frost of Contra Costa County. How can the best practices of some institutions and regions be developed into a national model?
- **Exercises and drills:** Participants repeatedly stressed the importance of drills and of exercising preparedness plans. Beyond practice, there also needs to be some level of competency. Speakers and participants called for national-level pediatric exercises and suggested that pediatric preparedness exercises should perhaps be a regulatory requirement for hospitals.
- **Workarounds versus safety and quality:** It was discussed that in the absence of feasible solutions to complex preparedness and response problems, workarounds are often developed. However, this raised concerns from a patient safety and quality of care

perspective. It was suggested that process engineers also be included in preparedness planning.

- **Disaster education:** While emergency preparedness is built on the strength of everyday health systems, professionals and the public should be better informed about their expected roles in a disaster, especially related to children. To be effective, pediatric training for providers must be built on comprehensive education and training in disaster management and emergency preparedness for all our nation's public health and health care providers, adult as well as pediatric. It must also ensure that pediatric-specific basic education and training in pediatric disaster management and emergency preparedness is offered not only to health care providers who have dedicated their professional lives to the care of children, but also to adult health care providers who in times of contingency or crisis may be called on to treat children until definitive pediatric care is available. Jeff Upperman presented innovative strategies on developing competencies in health care professionals, but more emphasis is needed both for providers and the general public on their role in disasters.
- **Lessons learned versus actions taken:** Disasters create moments of opportunity for advocacy and action. It is important to seize these moments when the public and policy makers are engaged to make change. Irwin Redlener of the National Center for Disaster Medicine and Public Health pointed out that lessons learned are nothing if they do not lead to action. Some suggested that after the near-steady stream of recent man-made and natural disasters and emergencies, the moment of opportunity is now.

2

Children and Disasters

Highlights of Points Made by Individual Speakers

- Many deficiencies exist in the data for preparedness planning related to children.
- The basic goal with respect to disasters is to make children, families, and communities more resilient and less vulnerable.
- Adults and children may initially persevere following a traumatic event, but the resilience can erode the longer recovery takes, and the more stressful the recovery process is over time.
- Progress continues to be made in the implementation of recommendations in 11 categories from the 2010 report authored by the National Commission on Children and Disasters.

This report begins with an overview of the specific impact of disasters on children by Irwin Redlener, director of the National Center for Disaster Preparedness at Columbia University. He explained the important differences between lessons learned and lessons acted on, and realistic goals to keep in mind regarding children in these precarious situations. This is followed by a review of the recommendations from the 2010 National Commission on Children in Disasters (NCCD) report and updates on progress being made in different sectors around the country.

NEEDED FOCUS ON CHILDREN AND FAMILIES

There are tremendous deficiencies in the data needed to plan appropriately for children, said keynote speaker Redlener, and as a population they do not have their own voice to use to their advantage. Children have very long memories, he continued, and the impact of the trauma associated with both the disaster itself, and prolonged or difficult recoveries, can last a very long time.

Lessons Learned Versus Actions Taken

People often look back at their experiences and call them "lessons learned." But Redlener highlighted the need to differentiate between something that happened, and something that happened that led to preventive actions to mitigate future adverse events. He offered several examples from the events that occurred between October 24, 2012, and May 31, 2013. During this 7-month period, there were 9 major incidents: Hurricane Sandy on the East Coast; the Sandy Hook Elementary School shooting in Newtown, Connecticut; bombings at the Boston Marathon; an explosion in a fertilizer plant in West, Texas; letters containing Ricin mailed to officials in Washington, DC; massive flooding in the Midwest; two EF5 tornadoes within 2 weeks in Moore and El Reno, Oklahoma; and a bridge collapse in Mount Vernon, Washington. Four of these incidents happened in 1 week, between Monday and Friday of April 15 through April 19 (Boston bombings, West explosion, DC Ricin letters, and Midwest flooding).

Children's Near Misses

Data are difficult to obtain, but it is estimated that across these 9 events there were 176 fatalities, 46 of which were children or adolescents (26 percent). Redlener also described some of the "close calls" in these events, situations that could have easily been far worse with respect to child injuries and fatalities. For example, during Hurricane Sandy, the New York University Langone Medical Center evacuated neonates from its neonatal intensive care unit. Photographs of people carrying tiny newborn babies down a dark hospital stairwell were front-page news. While evacuation helped to ensure continued intensive care, Redlener suggested that, had we learned from Hurricane Katrina and taken action to protect generators, fuel supplies, electrical systems, etc., there may not have been a need to move these delicate patients. In Boston, there happened to be very few children at the marathon finish line when the bombs detonated. What if, Redlener said, there had been a third-grade class watching the end of the marathon at that time? In West, Texas, the plant explosion caused extensive damage to the middle school and high school. Because the explosion happened after school hours, the middle school students were gone, and although the high school track team was returning to the school from an event, they decided to stop along the way for something to eat, delaying their return to school. Although hundreds of schools are in Oklahoma's "Tornado Alley" (most without appropriate storm cellars or other safe havens), the Moore, Oklahoma, tornado only destroyed one school (killing seven people in the school). In Mount Vernon, Washington, there were no children in the vehicles that plunged into the water when the bridge collapsed. Thankfully, there was not a school bus on the bridge at that time, he noted.

Turning Learning to Action

The questions, Redlener said, are what are we actually learning from these events and near misses, and how fast are we filling the gaps in preparedness and response that are identified? During only 215 days the country faced a hurricane superstorm, a school shooting, terrorism, an industrial accident, severe flooding, tornadoes, and infrastructure failure. Disasters are not going away. More severe weather is inevitable. Pandemic viruses continue to emerge. The country faces potential cyber attacks, nuclear plant meltdowns, improvised nuclear devices, chemical spills, earthquakes, and the list goes on.

Are we learning from these tragedies and close calls? For example, it is clear that children must be protected in schools. Alabama now requires newly built public schools to have adequate protection from tornadoes, but Redlener said he was not aware of any similar action in the Oklahoma State Legislature thus far. There is limited understanding about how to protect backup generators in hospitals. There is also a lack of preemptive evacuation protocols. Shelters, even those designated for families, are often ill prepared for children, lacking diapers, cribs, and baby food.

Recovery

Once the initial disaster event is over, it can take a very long time for a community to return to a normal level of functionality. When a community is at high risk for further disaster events, Redlener said, the goal is not to achieve the pre-event normal, but rather to achieve a new normal with better infrastructure and stability. Redlener referred to the recovery of infrastructure as "façade recovery." The buildings are rebuilt, the infrastructure is repaired, and there is the appearance of recovery. The recovery of the impacted population, however, takes much longer. He noted that surveys done 3, 5, and 7 years after Hurricane Katrina still indicated ongoing effects of the trauma.

Redlener also described the concept of "resilience erosion" (see Figure 2-1). People, including children, can initially persevere through a traumatic event. Children are buffered from stress by resilient adults who protect them through the period of trauma and recovery, and transmit a sense of resilience. However, the longer recovery takes, and the more stressful the recovery process is, the more difficult it is for the adult to remain a resilient buffer for the children. After weeks, months, and even years of waiting for the situation to improve, parents who were once strong begin to lose their ability to provide an emotional and functional safety net for their children. Adding to the stress is the lack of any central function that coordinates the various recovery assets available from federal, state, and local agencies, nonprofit organizations, the Red Cross, insurance companies, banks, and others. Instead, individuals who have been affected by the disaster must navigate the highly complex bureaucratic process on their own.

Setting and Achieving Goals

The basic goal with respect to disasters is to make children, families, and communities less vulnerable, and more resilient and safe. Toward this end, the 2010 NCCD report recommends specific actions to be taken to improve preparedness, response, and recovery for children (NCCD, 2010; discussed further by Schonfeld and Dodgen in the next section). In setting and achieving goals, there is what Redlener called a "denominator problem." If achievement is thought of as a fraction, what has been completed is the numerator and what is still needed is the denominator.

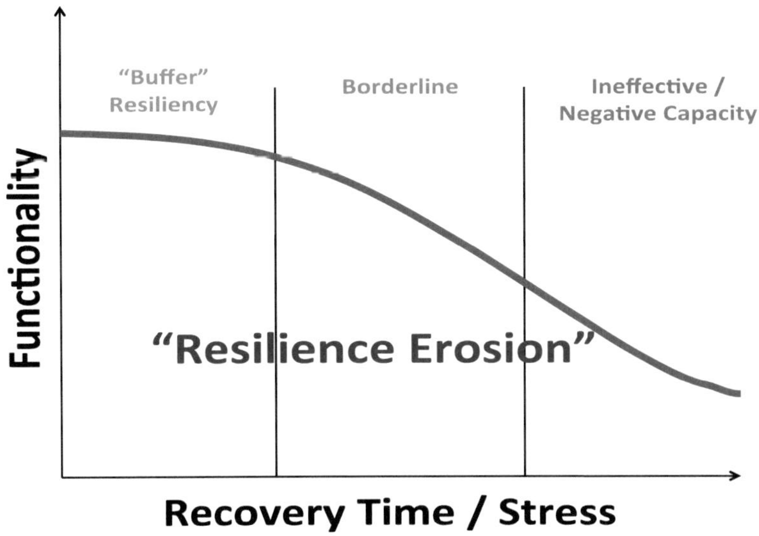

FIGURE 2-1 Resilience erosion.
SOURCE: Redlener presentation, June 10, 2013.

Government agencies are often interested in the numerator, and issue long lists of the progress that has been made. But the denominator of "continuing needs" is huge, he said, and because of this, children are still at risk. Through focusing more on the denominator—what is still left to be done—more needs can be identified.

There are definitely wins, Redlener stressed. There is leadership buy-in to the concept that children need to be protected, there is embedded pediatric expertise throughout government, and there are many advocates. But federalism and politics run counter to national disaster planning. Washington's priorities are not necessarily the end user's priorities, and it is the local governments who determine how and when they will spend money and what their priorities are. Further, the research base on children and disasters is insufficient, and preparedness and response funding continues to be cut. Redlener pointed out that in comparison to fiscal year (FY) 2010, the President's submitted budget for FY 2014 shows funding for the Hospital Preparedness Program (HPP) cut by 35 percent, state and local preparedness programs cut by 62 percent, and the elimination of the Academic and Public Health Preparedness Centers that had been promised a 5-year lifespan.

There are many community-based programs addressing preparedness. But Redlener suggested that the scale is too large to be handled solely on a local basis. High-functioning community-based models of children's preparedness are necessary, but are not replacements for government initiatives and large-scale funding.

In conclusion, Redlener said that with regard to children we should be hoping for the best and preparing for the worst, but given the economy, the political deadlock, and children's status among national priorities, we are instead hoping that we keep dodging the bullets.

2010 NATIONAL COMMISSION ON CHILDREN AND DISASTERS RECOMMENDATIONS

The NCCD 2010 *Report to the President and Congress*[1] provided recommendations in 11 major categories (see Appendix H). David Schonfeld, director of the National Center for School Crisis and Bereavement and former Commission member, shared his perspective on some of the progress made thus far in 8 of the 11 categories (omitting the last 3 due to time constraints).

Integration

The first NCCD recommendations on disaster management and recovery are really about integration, Schonfeld said. Recommendation 1.1 from the report is to "distinguish and comprehensively integrate the needs of children across all inter- and intra-governmental disaster management activities and operations." The recommendation specifies further that children should not be grouped in an "at-risk" category, but should instead be pulled out for separate consideration. Schonfeld listed several examples of how the needs of children are now being considered

---

[1]The National Commission on Children and Disasters was authorized under the Consolidated Appropriations Act of 2008, signed into law by President Bush on December 26, 2007 (P.L. 110-161). The Commission was charged with examining children's needs relative to disaster preparedness, response, and recovery, and the status of existing laws, regulations, policies, and programs relevant to meeting such needs. The final Commission findings and recommendations were delivered to President Obama and Congress in October 2010. The Commission was terminated in April 2011, per its charter. See http://www.ahrq.gov/prep/nccdreport for further information (accessed September 8, 2013).

in planning, response, and recovery efforts, including the establishment of children's working groups at the Federal Emergency Management Agency (FEMA) and Department of Health and Human Services (HHS), as well as significant focus on the needs of the children by the Centers for Disease Control and Prevention.

Recommendation 1.1 also specifies that "the Executive Branch at all levels of government should establish and maintain permanent focal points of coordination for children in disasters that are supported by sufficient authority, funding and policy expertise." Schonfeld said that significant progress has been made in incorporating pediatric subject-matter expertise and policy expertise. However, he noted that there are concerns about the permanence of these efforts and whether the experts actually do have sufficient authority to effect change on an ongoing basis. Of particular concern is the adequacy of funding. One opportunity to enhance integration comes under the Pandemic and All-Hazards Preparedness Act reauthorization, which calls for the establishment of a National Advisory Committee on Children in Disasters. According to Schonfeld, it is expected that this committee will have sufficient resources, support, and potential influence. But, as noted earlier by Anderson, there is uncertainty on where this committee will live, which reinforces the overall need for centralization for these issues and resources.

One gap in integration highlighted by the NCCD was the lack of inclusion of education, child care, juvenile justice, and child welfare systems into disaster planning, training, and exercises. Progress in this area has been hindered in large part by funding reductions. These partners are struggling to simply meet their core missions, and there is little to no supplemental funding to meet specific disaster preparedness response goals. If this is not remedied, Schonfeld said, much of the considerable progress that has been achieved stands to be lost.

Mental Health

Recommendation 2.1 in the report states that "HHS should lead efforts to integrate mental and behavioral health for children in public health, medical, and other relevant disaster management activities." Although there has been progress in this area, Schonfeld said that funding limitations have compromised the federal agencies and the non-federal partners' ability to enhance pre-disaster preparedness in pediatric disaster mental and behavioral health (e.g., psychological first aid, bereavement support, brief supportive interventions). Such preparedness training would be geared toward mental health professionals and other individuals who work with children (e.g., teachers). With regard to preparedness training, Schonfeld cautioned that "just-in-time" training is usually not in time. As an example, he described meeting with the school staff just after the shooting in Newtown, Connecticut. He observed that it was very difficult for the staff to process any information or training at that point.

Recommendation 2.4 calls for strengthening the Crisis Counseling Assistance and Training Program (CCP) to better meet the mental health needs of children and families. Schonfeld said that follow-up conversations (after the NCCD disbanded) with representatives of the CCP indicated that FEMA was generally in agreement with the changes recommended by the Commission, and was seeking mechanisms to implement them. Although overall progress toward successful implementation is not yet clear, there are some examples. Schonfeld cited the Crisis Counseling Grant awarded to New Jersey in response to Hurricane Sandy, which includes a community liaison, numerous children's specialists, and an intervention-based program to ensure that children's disaster mental health needs are addressed effectively and efficiently. Similar efforts are also under way in Oklahoma.

Child Physical Health and Trauma

Recommendation 3.1 calls on Congress, HHS, and the Department of Homeland Security (DHS)/FEMA to ensure the availability of and access to pediatric medical countermeasures. A recent Government Accountability Office report found that significant progress has been made in furthering the development of medical countermeasures (MCMs) for children; incorporating children's needs into planning at the state and local levels; and developing and distributing dosing and administration guidance materials for parents and other caregivers (GAO, 2013). There has also been attention to increasing the relative proportion of MCMs in the Strategic National Stockpile (SNS) that can be used for children. Pediatric experts now advise on the content of the SNS to ensure that pediatric needs are represented, and emergency use authorizations (EUAs) have been developed proactively so that stockpiling of MCMs used under EUAs is permitted. Despite this progress, challenges remain in the development, testing, and purchasing of sufficient pediatric MCMs. Most worrisome, Schonfeld suggested, is the erosion of funding to support the SNS, which threatens the ability to maintain even the current level of readiness in the SNS for pediatric MCMs.

Recommendations 3.2 and 3.3 advise HHS and the Department of Defense to enhance pediatric capabilities of their disaster medical response teams and to ensure that health professionals who may treat children during disasters have adequate pediatric disaster clinical training. In this regard, the National Disaster Medical System (NDMS)[2] has made significant efforts to increase the number of providers with pediatric expertise, but Schonfeld said that this effort by NDMS does not translate directly to comprehensive pediatric readiness in the field.

The NCCD also recommended establishing a formal regionalized pediatric system of care to support pediatric surge capacity during and after disasters. Schonfeld highlighted the NCCD's concern that the country is not yet prepared to accommodate a surge in pediatric emergency medical trauma that may occur during a disaster, although, as of yet, no North American emergency to date has overwhelmed intensive care unit services on a widespread basis since the modern development of the field of critical care. However, planners are not optimistic that this will always be the case, and important progress on Pediatric Emergency Mass Critical Care has been made in recent years (Kissoon, 2011).

Another recommendation in this area calls for prioritizing the recovery of pediatric health and mental health care delivery systems in disaster affected areas. There has been no progress in establishing a funding mechanism to support the restoration and continuity of for-profit health and mental health services for children, and this remains a significant vulnerability, Schonfeld said.

---

[2]The NDMS is a federally coordinated system to provide disaster medical care to the nation. The mission of NDMS is to "temporarily supplement federal, tribal, state and local capabilities by funding, organizing, training, equipping, deploying and sustaining a specialized and focused range of public health and medical capabilities." For further information, see http://www.phe.gov/preparedness/responders/ndms/Pages/default.aspx (accessed September 9, 2013).

Emergency Medical Services and Pediatric Transport

Recommendation 4.1 states that "the President and Congress should clearly designate and appropriately resource a lead federal agency for emergency medical services with primary responsibility for the coordination of grant programs, research, policy, and standards development and implementation." Although Schonfeld opined that this remains a need not only for disaster preparedness, but also for optimizing routine pediatric emergency medical services across the country, this view may not be uniformly shared across the emergency medical services (EMS) community. Given that EMS interfaces with so many different federal agencies, creating one federal lead may not solve issues that reach across so many areas.

Schonfeld described the commission's call for efforts to "improve the capability of emergency medical services to transport pediatric patients and provide comprehensive pre-hospital pediatric care during daily operations and disasters," and to "develop a national strategy to improve federal pediatric emergency transport and patient care capabilities for disasters." The limited federal and state capability to accommodate a major pediatric surge requiring transport of a large number of pediatric patients is a significant vulnerability.

Disaster Case Management

The single recommendation in this area, Section 5, states that "disaster case management programs should be appropriately resourced and should provide consistent holistic services that achieve tangible positive outcomes for children and families affected by disasters." Further, "government agencies and NGOs [nongovernmental organizations] should develop voluntary consensus standards on the essential elements and methods of disaster case management including pre-credentialing of case managers and training that includes focused attention to the needs of children and families." Case management of a family is much more than making sure they have a place to live temporarily, Schonfeld explained.

To this end, the Administration for Children and Families (ACF) is developing a model of case management that provides more comprehensive services and addresses the needs of children and families more appropriately.[3] Schonfeld noted, however, that these standards have not yet been broadly adopted.

Child Care and Early Education

In Section 6, the NCCD recommended that "Congress and HHS should improve disaster preparedness capabilities for child care," including requiring states to include disaster planning, training, and exercising within the scope of minimum health and safety standards for child care licensure or registration, and requiring Head Start Centers to have disaster preparedness capabilities and to provide basic disaster mental health training for their staff.[4]

There is some growing interest in disaster preparedness among Head Start Programs. Schonfeld cited as an example a recent workshop sponsored by the American Academy of Pediatrics at the Head Start Leadership Institute in Washington, DC. In addition, ACF issued a proposed regulation that would require emergency preparedness and response planning for providers serving children who are receiving child care development fund assistance. Such planning would include provisions for evacuation and relocation, sheltering in place, and family reunification. Despite these efforts, most of the recommendations in this section have not yet been implemented, and the state of readiness of child care in early education is a major gap, Schonfeld said. The ongoing concern is that schools, child care, and early education centers are not sufficiently prepared to recover promptly from natural disasters and they remain potential soft but high-impact targets for terrorism.

Elementary and Secondary Education

Moving to Section 7 of the NCCD report, Schonfeld conveyed the commission's concerns about the limited funds available to improve the preparedness of schools and school districts. The recommendations in this section call for DHS and FEMA to partner with the Department of

---

[3]Update: *The Disaster Case Management Concept of Operations* is now online; see http://www.acf.hhs.gov/programs/ohsepr/disaster-case-management (accessed November 1, 2013).

[4]The *Head Start Emergency Preparedness Manual* can be found at http://eclkc.ohs.acf.hhs.gov/hslc/tta-system/health/ep (accessed November 1, 2013).

Education to provide additional "funding and other resources to support disaster preparedness efforts of state and local education agencies, including collaborative planning, training, and exercises with emergency management officials." The commission also called for funding to states to "implement and evaluate training and professional development programs in basic skills in providing support to grieving students and students in crisis, and to establish state-wide requirements related to teacher certification and recertification" in these areas.

The Readiness for Emergency Management in Schools (REMS) program was highlighted by the NCCD as a worthwhile mechanism for delivering grant funding to school districts for preparedness that should be expanded. However, funding for the REMS grant programs has been eliminated, and Schonfeld noted that there has been little progress toward the goal of implementing or evaluating the training and professional development of educators and other school personnel. At a recent White House event on school preparedness that was held after the school shooting in Newtown, Connecticut, there was a clear call from partners to reverse the cuts to the REMS grant program and to expand it substantially, as called for by the NCCD. Unfortunately, Schonfeld said, this is one area where ground has been lost, rather than progress made, and school systems and their students remain unprepared to deal with disasters, whether natural or man-made.

> "School systems and their students remain unprepared to deal with disasters, whether natural or man-made."
> —David J. Schonfeld

Child Welfare and Juvenile Justice

The NCCD made several recommendations aimed at ensuring that state and local child welfare agencies, juvenile justice agencies (and their associated court programs), and residential treatment, correctional, and detention facilities that house children become adequately prepared for disasters to minimize the impact of these events and to support rapid recovery. Recommendations 8.1, 8.2, and 8.3 call for an evaluation of current status; issuing of planning guidance; provision of funding, guidance, and technical assistance; and the establishment of minimal standards of preparedness. Schonfeld said that there has been some review of current preparedness, and the Department of Justice is preparing a pilot competitive grant program to states to support the development of emergency preparedness plans for juvenile justice facilities. Still, there has not yet been sufficient response to remedy the gap as called for by the NCCD.

Sheltering, Housing, and Evacuation

The remaining three groups of recommendations in Sections 9, 10, and 11 address sheltering standards, services, and supplies; housing, including prioritizing the needs of families with children (including those with children who have disabilities or chronic physical or mental health needs) in temporary and long-term disaster housing; and evacuation, including reunification of children with their families after disasters.

HHS PROGRESS IN ADDRESSING CHILDREN'S DISASTER HEALTH NEEDS

The NCCD recommendations directed toward HHS fall into four key categories: behavioral health; MCMs; physical health, EMS, and transport; and child care and child welfare. To address these, ACF and the Office of the Assistant Secretary for Preparedness and Response (ASPR) established the Children's HHS Interagency Leadership on Disasters (CHILD) Working Group comprised of members from 18 HHS divisions. The working group was created to comprehensively integrate the disaster-related health and human services needs of children across HHS disaster policy, planning, and operations activities; to assess current capabilities and facilitate coordination at the policy and response levels; and to develop a set of recommendations to enhance departmental efforts (see Box 2-1). An overview of progress by HHS in the four areas was provided by Dan Dodgen, director of the Division for At-Risk Individuals, Behavioral Health, and Community Resilience in ASPR.[5]

---

[5]Dodgen referred participants to the Division for At-Risk Individuals, Behavioral Health, and Community Resilience website for further information: http://www.phe.gov/abc (accessed September 9, 2013).

Behavioral Health

Dodgen highlighted some of the key accomplishments thus far in the area of behavioral health, noting that these actions were taken in response to both the recommendations of the NCCD and recommendations of the National BioDefense Science Board.

BOX 2-1
Children's Health and Human Services Interagency Leadership on Disasters (CHILD) Working Group Recommendations for Health and Human Services Action

<u>Behavioral Health</u>

- Develop and implement a concept of operations for disaster behavioral health.
- Implement internal, programmatic improvements to the Crisis Counseling Assistance and Training Program (CCP).
- Leverage new/expanded health home and behavioral health benefits authorized by the Affordable Care Act (ACA) to promote health and resilience in children.
- Update HHS grants to improve integration among public health, behavioral health, and health care delivery systems.
- Enhance the research agenda for children's disaster mental health.
- Promote and disseminate just-in-time training on children's mental health for caregivers, professionals, and responders.

<u>Medical Countermeasures (MCMs)</u>

- Establish an integrated program team to advise the Public Health Emergency Medical Counter Measures Enterprise (PHEMCE) on pediatric and obstetric (OB) MCM priorities.
- Incorporate pediatric and OB-specific vulnerabilities in scenario and medical consequence modeling for requirements.
- Provide clarity in the regulatory pathway for pediatric MCMs (e.g., stockpiling, forward deployment, clinical guidance).
- Engage the pediatric MCM community on a regular basis.
- Continue and improve industry support for research and development of MCMs suitable to pediatric use.
- Include pediatric and OB expertise in the Public Health Emergency Research Review Board (PHERRB) to support data collection for assessing safety and efficacy of MCMs.

Physical Health, Emergency Medical Services (EMS), Transport

- Evaluate the recruitment and deployment process of the National Disaster Medical System Multi-Specialty Enhancement Team.
- Strengthen requirements for pediatric surge capacity within the Health Care Preparedness Program (HPP) and encourage HHS grantees to adopt the Emergency Medical Services for Children (EMSC) pediatric equipment list for ambulances and other guidelines.
- Take a lead role in setting educational and operational standards for pre-hospital care, particularly for children.
- Convene stakeholders to assess capabilities and address gaps for large-scale pediatric patient movement.
- Train NDMS personnel in pediatric disaster medicine to ensure basic clinical skills.

Child Care and Child Welfare

- Implement and promote the Administration for Children and Families (ACF) Information Memorandum that provides guidance to Child Care and Development Fund Lead Agencies in developing, exercising, and maintaining comprehensive emergency preparedness and response plans for child care.
- Develop a cross-regional review of child welfare disaster plans to identify strengths, areas for improvement, and targeted technical assistance.
- Make available additional outreach and training efforts for states to increase their understanding of the Disaster Case Management program.
- Ensure children and others with access and functional needs are included in relevant disaster services trainings.

SOURCE: Dodgen presentation, June 10, 2013.

First, HHS created and implemented a Disaster Behavioral Health Concept of Operations[6] designed to provide coordination and guidance for federal-level behavioral response. As a result, children's behavioral health is now part of every HHS response and recovery to disasters. For example, HHS provided support in response to the Newtown, Connecticut, shooting, Hurricane Sandy, and the Joplin tornadoes through the

[6]The HHS Disaster Behavioral Health Concept of Operations is available at http://www.phe.gov/Preparedness/planning/abc/Documents/dbh-conops.pdf (accessed September 9, 2013).

CCP, which sent trained crisis counselors into the community and schools to work with children.

To build capacity, ASPR leadership and NDMS responders have been trained in psychological first aid, the U.S. Public Health Service Commissioned Corps includes psychological first aid in all of its field training activities, and a 6-hour, interactive, online psychological first aid course available through National Child Traumatic Stress Network.[7]

In 2012, the Substance Abuse and Mental Health Services Administration (SAMHSA) launched the Disaster Distress Helpline (DDH), the first hotline dedicated to providing disaster crisis counseling. The DDH offers support via telephone and Short Message Service (SMS) text, and hosted a Twitter chat on helping children and teenagers cope after disasters. The line is always active and ready for use, Dodgen explained, and capacity can be increased as events happens. Dodgen commended SAMHSA for making the disaster distress line readily accessible via forms of communication that are popular among adolescents (e.g., texting and Twitter).

Medical Countermeasures

We are beginning to make some real strides in moving forward the MCM enterprise for children, Dodgen said. For example, a pediatric and obstetric integrated program team was established to provide guidance to PHEMCE and prioritize gaps related to pediatric and obstetrical needs. There are now a number of pediatric MCM initiatives under way. In May 2013, for example, the Biomedical Advanced Research and Development Authority (BARDA) awarded a contract for the development of the antibiotic solithromycin for the treatment of children infected with anthrax, tularemia, or community-acquired bacterial pneumonia. Clinical studies have also been funded by the National Institutes of Health and BARDA to support a pediatric indication for midazolam to treat nerve-agent seizures, and they should be widely distributed within stockpiles for children once approved. Though, as benzodiazepines (midazolam family) are commonly used for the treatment of seizure disorders in children, clinical studies on drugs that are not used as often or where effects are less clear could also be illuminating. In addition, the National Institute of Child Health and Human Development Pediatric Trials

[7]The psychological first aid course is available at http://learn.nctsn.org/course/category.php?id=11 (accessed September 9, 2013).

Network plans to conduct 16 trials in the next 5 years that could enhance pediatric labeling of MCMs. There are also activities aimed at addressing the unique challenges of developing MCMs for children. For example, the U.S. Food and Drug Administration held a public workshop on the Ethical and Regulatory Challenges in the Development of Pediatric Medical Countermeasures.

Physical Health, EMS, and Transport

Dodgen highlighted several accomplishments in the areas of pediatric physical health, EMS, and transport. The NDMS has developed the capability to deploy pediatric specialists to augment traditional response teams. The intent is to have people with unique expertise who may not need to respond to every emergency setting, but who are available when needed. To help address pediatric patient movement, ASPR hosted two workshops with pediatric transport stakeholders and additional workshops are planned. To aid reunification, one outcome of the Pediatric Disaster Preparedness Curriculum Development Conference convened by the National Center for Disaster Medicine and Public Health was an online module, "Tracking and Reunification of Children in Disasters: A Lesson and Reference for Health Professionals."[8] The ASPR HPP hosted a technical assistance webinar in June 2013 for HPP grantees and health care coalitions on integrating pediatric disaster management into health care system preparedness and medical surge.[9] Approximately 400 people dialed in to participate in the webinar, and the archived webpage received 3,000 visits in the first month it was available. A second webinar focused on pediatrics is scheduled for May 2014 through the HPP at ASPR.

These are just a few examples of current programs, and Dodgen noted that the goal is not to simply create more federal mechanisms and federal projects, but to involve the stakeholders and people at the local level who will ultimately implement the programs.

---

[8]Module is available at http://ncdmph.usuhs.edu/KnowledgeLearning/2012-Learning1.htm (accessed September 9, 2013).

[9]The webinar is archived at http://www.phe.gov/Preparedness/planning/abc/Pages/webinar-resources-130620.aspx (accessed September 9, 2013) along with all of the resources identified, from both federal agencies and nongovernment partners.

Child Care and Child Welfare

There is a lot of activity on child care and child welfare happening at ACF right now, Dodgen said. For example, ACF has trained all of the nation's State Administrators for Family Violence Prevention and Services on disaster preparedness, including attention to the needs of children exposed to domestic violence. ACF has also trained Head Start executives in preparedness planning. ACF recently collaborated with state and NGO partners via Child Care Task Forces and Coalitions following the Joplin tornadoes and Hurricanes Isaac and Sandy to assess the impacts to systems serving children and to promote children's resilience and recovery. (Efforts toward improved child and family welfare during disaster recovery are discussed further in Chapter 8.)

Next Steps for HHS

HHS has been responsive to the recommendations of the Commission and other stakeholders, and has covered a lot of the basic areas, Dodgen said, but there is still work to be done. The CHILD working group has prioritized three additional areas of focus for 2012-2013: children with special health care needs and other subpopulations of children traditionally under-represented in planning efforts; pregnant/breastfeeding women and neonates; and enhancing inter-departmental and NGO collaboration. The working group plans to submit its second progress report to HHS leadership at the end of 2013. In closing, Dodgen said that Assistant Secretary Lurie and ASPR are committed to ensuring that children are integrated into all emergency preparedness, response, and recovery efforts. HHS policies and programs will continue to emphasize and address the disaster health and human services needs of children and families. He stressed that, in the face of the sequester budget challenges, there is no longer room for isolated projects. Collaboration across federal agencies and with outside stakeholders is essential.

3

Leveraging Health Care Coalitions

Highlights of Points Made by Individual Speakers

- Pediatric surge capacity remains a challenge.
- Barriers to building capability include lack of understanding among stakeholders of each other's needs and capabilities, lack of local knowledge about available guidance and tools, and cost.
- A coalition's role is translating across silos, promoting day-to-day pediatric readiness, helping communities navigate through numerous disaster preparedness tools, and partnering to make the best use of available resources.
- National neonatal and pediatric disaster drills are needed.

This chapter focuses on how best to leverage existing coalitions and collaborations for the benefit of children. Panelists provided federal, state, and local perspectives on coalition challenges and best practices, and discussed duality of services and improving everyday capacity. Securing buy-in from important stakeholders and coordinating work across regions and sectors are a few of the challenges discussed, as well as highlighting the need for central coordination and broadening of stakeholders in coalitions past simply including pediatric providers.

Giving an example of ways to augment pediatric surge capacity, Andrew Rucks of the University of Alabama at Birmingham noted that he also serves as director of the Southeastern Regional Pediatric Disaster Surge Network, which currently includes Alabama, Florida, Georgia, Louisiana, Mississippi, and Tennessee, and will soon include Kentucky, North Carolina, and South Carolina. The network is an emerging multistate coalition of health departments, children's specialty hospitals, regional hospitals, emergency responders, first responders, and local community pediatricians who are coming together to provide surge capacity in a region of the country that has very limited surge capacity to deal with children. The network has developed a mission and is working to operationalize and exercise the surge network, pointing to an earlier referenced challenge about the lack of pediatric focused exercises and drills. There are numerous challenges to managing this multistate coalition consisting of a wide variety of players, Rucks said. And while regions are becoming better prepared to deal with large-scale events (e.g., hurricanes), Rucks suggested that they are not as well prepared to deal with the smaller-scale issues that overwhelm the needs of one or more local pediatric specialty hospitals.

FEDERAL PERSPECTIVE: THE HOSPITAL PREPAREDNESS PROGRAM

Richard Hunt, senior medical advisor for the National Health Care Preparedness Programs at the Office of the Assistant Secretary for Preparedness and Response (ASPR), provided federal-level perspective on health care coalitions. Currently, the U.S. health care delivery system is focused on cost reduction. This includes service retraction, which results in just-in-time operating principles and staffing. Although U.S. health systems emergency preparedness and response mechanisms are established and operational, they are fragmented and are restrained by a just-in-time approach, Hunt said. The country continues to experience overcrowding in emergency departments with limited mechanisms to reallocate patients throughout the hospital or the community. Although the concept of surge capacity has been discussed for well over a decade, a March 2013 Government Accountability Office report still highlights surge capacity as a challenge. Work has been done on allocation of scarce resources and introducing the concept of crisis standards of care, where population outcomes would be optimized over individual patient outcomes (Devereaux et al., 2008; IOM, 2012). Although this difficult conversation is further complicated when children are introduced to the discussion, it is an important piece in planning if a scenario occurred where real limitations were placed on resources or capabilities.

Hunt described some of the financial realities of disaster preparedness and response. National health care expenditures grew 4 percent to $2.5 trillion in 2009, or $8,086 per person, and accounted for 17.6 percent of gross domestic product. Hospital expenditures for 2010 were $814 billion according to the Centers for Medicare & Medicaid Services. Assuming there were 5,754 hospitals in the United States (per the American Hospital Association), the average hospital expenditure was approximately $141 million that year. In contrast, the total Hospital Preparedness Program (HPP) budget for 2012 was $347 million, which Hunt pointed out is 0.0001 percent of overall national health expenditures.

With that in mind, Hunt said, the current need is a comprehensive national preparedness and response health care system that is scalable and coordinated to meet local, state, and national needs, and is financially sustainable. This requires a multifaceted effort, including integrating with and improving the efficiency of daily health care delivery, and applying a population-based health care–delivery model for disaster response. Toward that end, having defined health care preparedness capabilities (i.e., goals) and performance measures is very important.

Fifteen capabilities for national health care preparedness are outlined by ASPR in the National Guidance for Health care System Preparedness (ASPR, 2012). Health care system preparedness is one area where HPP is currently focusing efforts. Hunt described health care coalition development as the foundation for health care preparedness capabilities. The concept is one of inclusiveness, like a web, where the whole is greater than the sum of its parts. Per the ASPR guidance, the list of health care coalition essential partner memberships includes "specialty service providers (e.g., dialysis, pediatrics, women's health, stand-alone surgery, urgent care)." It will be important moving forward for pediatrics to interface with coalitions, and for pediatric coalitions to interface with the health care preparedness program. Hunt noted that the Pediatric Preparedness Resource Kit[1] released by the American Academy of Pediatrics includes an entire section on pediatric coalitions.

Hunt described four key considerations for developing a preparedness and response coalition. First, the coalition must be functional (i.e., not simply a mechanism for further discussions). Second, it is important to consider the percent of the population covered in a particular area relative to resources (e.g., how a very rural coalition

---

[1]Available at http://www.aap.org/en-us/advocacy-and-policy/aap-health-initiatives/Children-and-Disasters/Documents/PedPreparednessKit.pdf (accessed September 9, 2013).

compares to one that covers a much larger percentage of the population). The third consideration is the necessary linkage of preparedness with daily delivery of health care. Finally, risk needs to be taken into account. One aspect of risk could be, for example, how many coalitions cover a particular earthquake fault line? But another risk consideration is vulnerable or at-risk populations (e.g., older adults and children). Hunt stressed that ASPR is committed to building functional coalitions for national health care preparedness that not only work, but that will serve children as well.

LOCAL PERSPECTIVE: THE CALIFORNIA NEONATAL/PEDIATRIC DISASTER COALITION

Patricia Frost, director of Emergency Medical Services (EMS) for Contra Costa County Health Services in California, described a local, grassroots coalition-building effort and how coalitions can help overcome barriers to pediatric disaster preparedness. Contra Costa County in California has a population of 1.1 million, with about 250,000 children. A 2008 EMS for Children Program Assessment revealed that the county has lost more than 40 percent of its total pediatric bed capacity in the prior 5 years, and had approximately 1 licensed pediatric bed for every 16,000 children in Contra Costa. No one knew or considered the impact of this to the health system, she said.

> "In most communities across the nation, less than four to five critical pediatric patients, per hospital, arriving on the same day would completely saturate the pediatric health care system in that community."
>
> —Patricia Frost

A primary barrier to building capability, according to Frost, is the lack of understanding among stakeholders of each other's needs and capabilities. Frost observed that many times what one group perceives as simply excuses from another are, in fact, real barriers for them. A major role for a coalition is to translate across the gaps and silos, and to help find workarounds for complex problems.

Frost described the 2009 H1N1 influenza pandemic as a "pediatric disaster near miss" that helped launch the California Neonatal/Pediatric Disaster Coalition.[2] The first challenge for the grassroots effort to

[2]Frost referred participants to the coalition's GoogleSite, https://sites.google.com/site/pedineonetwork and the Contra Costa Pediatric Disaster Preparedness Resources website,

enhance pediatric capacity was to get people's attention. The coalition addressed this by telling a compelling story about the lack of licensed pediatric beds in the state. The state had never done a bed capacity analysis for neonatal and pediatrics, citing lack of funding. Frost found that California and the West Coast's pediatric "safety net" consists of about eight key regional centers that handle more than 55 percent of pediatric inpatient care. Every one of these is on a fault line at high risk for earthquakes. If, for example, Southern California lost its infrastructure for neonatal intensive care, providers may have to look as far as Texas to find bed capacity.

Another role of the coalition is to promote a strategic plan to improve day-to-day pediatric readiness. We need to plan for those situations that fall in between daily triage, when resources are available relative to patient demand and normal standards of care are applied, and full-scale disaster, when patient needs outstrip resources and crisis standards of care come into play. It does not take much to overwhelm the current system of pediatric care, Frost said. According to her experience, in most communities across the nation, less than four to five critical pediatric patients, per hospital, arriving on the same day would completely saturate the pediatric health care system in that community.

Lack of local knowledge about available guidance and tools is another barrier to preparedness. The coalition's role is the navigator through numerous (often overlapping) disaster preparedness tools, helping communities understand what they need to prepare for and how. With regard to tools, Frost also advocated for the use of communication technology under normal conditions. The goal is to embed technology, telemedicine, and consultation into normal pediatric care because it builds relationships and competencies. This knowledge, shared now, pays dividends when the power is lost later.

Cost is an ongoing barrier to preparedness. The coalition's role is not to raise money for itself, but rather to partner with organizations that have resources, and to direct communities to the training and other resources already available for free.[3] In addition, although hospitals are often competitors in a business sense, they must "share without regard to turf" when it comes to readiness.

---

http://cchealth.org/ems/emsc-disaster-prepare.php, for further information (accessed September 9, 2013).

[3]Frost cited, for example, the University of New Mexico Pediatric Emergency Online Education Program, available at http://hsc.unm.edu/emermed/PED/education onlineEd.shtml (accessed September 9, 2013).

Competency requires volume, and everyone can make a contribution, Frost said. The role of the coalition is to help set reasonable expectations, and craft messages to reduce fear. “Special” may be interpreted as “too scary to handle” for a community hospital, and adult providers may lack confidence in dealing with pediatric patients. Coalitions, both formal and informal, mobilize partners, and small collective actions matter. The California Neonatal/Pediatric Disaster Coalition has grown from a handful of key people to more than 150 champions statewide.

Frost concluded noting that we are very good at multi-agency and organization mobilization to save one or several children (for example, the rescue of 18-month-old Jessica McClure when she fell 22 feet down an 8-inch-wide well in 1987), but we tend to lose our focus when many more children are involved. Frost suggested that the next priority for the HPP should be a national neonatal and pediatric disaster drill. This, she said, could be the single most important vehicle to improve capability.

HOSPITAL PERSPECTIVE: NEW YORK CITY PEDIATRIC DISASTER COALITION

On the evening of Saturday, May 1, 2010, a sports utility vehicle packed with explosives was parked near Times Square in New York City, across the street from the theater where the family musical *The Lion King* was playing. The bomb failed, but had it exploded, there would likely have been numerous children in the area. George Foltin, vice chair of clinical services at Maimonides Infant and Children’s Hospital, described a study conducted by the New York City Pediatric Disaster Coalition to determine how many pediatric intensive care unit (PICU) beds were available in New York City on that day at that time. Although New York has a very sustainable and robust health care system and many pediatric intensive care beds, on that night only 21 percent of the pediatric beds were available, or 32 total beds. This potential disaster, paired with the bed census study, demonstrates the need to develop pediatric critical care surge capacity to increase the number of available beds in an emergency.

Coalition-Developed Resources

During the past decade, there has been a strong coalition between the New York City Department of Health and the health care sector. Because there are now hospitals focused exclusively on children, general hospitals have probably done the least thus far to prepare for children. Foltin cited as an example the 2008 development of guidelines to help hospitals prepare to receive children in a disaster. The resource guides general hospitals on elements such as security, how to put a baby in an adult bed, what kind of food and how much should be provided for children, and so forth. A pediatric disaster tabletop exercise was also developed to help hospitals exercise their plans.[4] Another resource the New York coalition developed for out-of-hospital pediatric disaster preparedness describes the elements of disaster planning and management for pre-hospital providers.[5]

The New York City Department of Health and Mental Hygiene also directed federal funds for a formalized Pediatric Disaster Coalition of hospitals, public health entities, municipal services, and community groups. The coalition is focused on effectively matching critical assets and resources to victim's needs during and after a large-scale disaster affecting children, neonates, and women in labor. The coalition will also develop and expand ongoing pediatric disaster preparedness efforts through advisory and coalition-building activities.

> "Major pediatric centers must be able to surge as critically ill children are best served at specialty centers."
>
> —George Foltin

Continuing to describe resources his coalition has developed, Foltin explained that a child's chances of survival are heavily dependent on the early chain of events, including triage, tiering, and transport (e.g., whether the child gets access to pediatric expertise right away, or whether they receive interim treatment at a facility not set up to handle children, followed by transport elsewhere). To help address this, the Pediatric Disaster Coalition created new guidelines for first responders, recommending transport of pediatric patients to pediatric receiving hospitals. A memorandum of understanding was established with the fire

[4]The hospital guidelines and the tabletop exercise toolkit are available at http://www.nyc.gov/html/doh/html/em/emergency-ped.shtml (accessed September 9, 2013).

[5]Available at http://cpem.med.nyu.edu/teaching-materials/pediatric-disaster-preparedness (accessed September 9, 2013).

department and EMS for inter-hospital transport after a disaster, because children may not have been initially transported to pediatric receiving hospitals. Pediatric intensive care surge plans were also developed, increasing pediatric surge bed capacity by an additional 128 beds above the baseline of 238. The coalition also worked with EMS to modify their triage process for children, and developed proposed hospital triage tiers for pediatric disaster victim transport based on pediatric capability of hospitals relative to the pediatric population (see Figure 3-1).

Foltin mentioned the Pediatric Fundamental Critical Care Support curriculum developed by the Society for Critical Care Medicine as one resource for hospitals to train providers in pediatric care during a disaster.[6] Other coalition activities Foltin mentioned include pediatric tabletop and full-scale exercises of PICU Surge Plans, activities focused on neonatal and maternal health, and a working group to study the successes and gaps in the pediatric response to Hurricane Sandy.

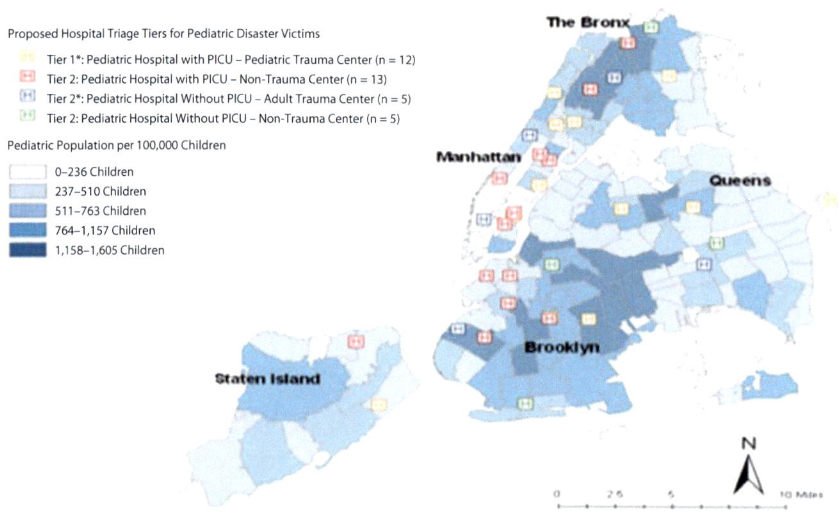

FIGURE 3-1 Proposed hospital triage tiers for pediatric disaster victims mapped against pediatric population density.
NOTE: PICU = pediatric intensive care unit.
SOURCE: Foltin presentation, June 10, 2013, citing Dana Meranus, New York City Department of Health and Mental Hygiene, April 2009.

[6]Available at http://www.sccm.org/Fundamentals/PFCCS/Pages/default.aspx (accessed September 9, 2013).

In conclusion, there must be a plan and communication, Foltin said. Major pediatric centers must be able to surge as critically ill children are best served at specialty centers. Primary transport should be to these centers, and inter-hospital transportation must be in place for children initially transported elsewhere. If this is not possible, general hospitals that are used to serving adults should have plans in place to properly take care of children. Building on just planning, resources, and drills are essential, he noted. Providers who do not routinely care for children often do not understand the subtleties, and many are very intimidated by it. If we do not prepare providers for the challenges and horrors of taking care of large numbers of badly injured children, they will not be able to care for the children successfully (or for adults, or even for themselves).

4

Augmenting State and Local Emergency Plans

Highlights of Points Made by Individual Speakers

- Pediatricians play a unique role in the health of children and families. Engaging community medical practices in preparedness efforts is essential to building community resilience.
- A systems-based approach is needed to ensure that stakeholders are preparing in the context of other partners in the community, and not in isolation.
- Individual parents and children who experience quarantine or isolation may need behavioral health and other support services to prevent or mitigate traumatic effects from social distancing.
- State and local preparedness and response plans including pandemics should include a module of pediatric health and mental/behavioral health.
- Bringing in stakeholders and adapting other state resources were key points in Illinois' development of a pediatric annex to their state emergency plan.

In order to adequately integrate the needs of children and their families into state and local emergency plans, it is necessary to involve those groups that represent different populations, as well as use best practices or evidence-informed guidelines. This section of the report brings together identified needs of children and families and discusses how to integrate them into municipal emergency plans. Several examples of issues, including pandemic planning and behavioral impacts, pediatric surge planning, and child care provider issues are discussed to help augment the material that goes into plans.

PROVIDER PERSPECTIVE: INTEGRATING COMMUNITY PEDIATRIC PRACTICES INTO DISASTER PREPAREDNESS

Esther Chernak of Drexel University School of Public Health described the development of a strategic plan to integrate pediatric practices into community-wide disaster preparedness. A systems-based approach helped to ensure that practices were prepared in the context of other partners in the community. The project was conducted by Drexel University in partnership with the Pennsylvania chapter of the American Academy of Pediatrics (PA AAP) and was funded by the Pennsylvania Department of Health through a Centers for Disease Control and Prevention Cooperative Agreement.

The primary objectives of the project were to identify the current status and needs of pediatric providers in the community with respect to emergency preparedness; identify the expectations of health departments; and formulate recommendations to improve the integration and coordination of pediatric providers. In conducting the project, it was assumed that physicians play a key role in promoting personal preparedness and in risk communications to the public (Garrett et al., 2007; Lasker, 2004; Olympia et al., 2010). It was also assumed that practice-level planning and outreach was important to realize the potential of practices, and that working with pediatric practices would be a paradigm for other primary care providers in the community.

The process was informed by a literature review and interviews with thought leaders and stakeholders in pediatrics, public health, emergency management, information technology, human services, health insurance, and schools/child care. The findings, Chernak noted, were not surprising. Most pediatricians had limited understanding of the public health system (e.g., how the agencies are organized, and their capacity, operations, and resources). They wanted a clear identification of their roles in a disaster, and felt that they had subject-matter expertise to share (e.g., pediatrics, understanding of public fears). Many providers simply do not have the time (or interest) in preparedness planning, but they were very interested in a just-in-time infrastructure for training during a disaster. They want real-time, pediatric-specific information to be able to ensure the continuity of operations and communicate with patients. Importantly, pediatricians want information before the public receives it, so that when patients call, they can speak knowledgeably about the issues and impacts.

It was also found that public health departments had a very limited understanding of pediatric practices, including how providers might function in public health emergencies. They failed to recognize the potential of pediatricians for disaster communications during an incident, and overestimated the capacity for outpatient practices to surge. Readiness has been very focused on points of dispensing (PODs) and mass prophylaxis in the first 48 hours of a disaster, with little planning for what happens after the POD closes. Public health departments also do not have an understanding of where practices are with regard to implementation of electronic records, including the potential and challenges of electronic health records (EHRs).

The first action, in collaboration with stakeholders, was to define the roles and expectations. For most pediatricians, their major role is in their community-based office, providing all aspects of medical care. This offsets the burden on hospitals, particularly emergency departments, Chernak noted. They also support the medical countermeasure enterprise, not just by staffing a POD, but by monitoring for drug interactions, adverse events, and outcomes after the POD closes. Providers also have a role in long-term follow-up and mental health support. Key roles for public health departments include local and state leadership, surveillance and investigation, implementation of disease control measures, surge support, and information sharing.

The project then developed recommendations for public health departments, pediatricians, and the PA AAP in the areas of continuity of operations and surge capacity building; collaborative planning; bi-directional communications; training; children with special health care needs; and schools and child care programs. Chernak highlighted several of the recommendations that she said were most relevant to health care coalitions (see Box 4-1).

Chernak referred participants to a recently released communications tool for pediatric practices[1] that includes fact sheet templates for waiting rooms and websites, phone scripts for voicemail and patient messaging, triage protocols, and social media templates. The PA AAP has been reaching out through webinars addressing continuity of operations and practices, mental health issues, and children with special health care needs, and is developing a list of pediatric subject-matter experts who can serve as advisors on an ad hoc basis to county health departments and the state health department.

---

[1]Available at https://www.portal.state.pa.us/portal/server.pt/document/1337530/final aap_toolkit_5_2_13_.pdf (accessed September 9, 2013).

BOX 4-1
Pennsylvania Strategic Plan Recommendations

Collaborative Planning

- Create a Pennsylvania Child Health Advisory Council for Disasters.
    - Include key stakeholders from across the Commonwealth such as practices, hospitals, schools, child care programs, government agencies.
    - Include a "rapid response" component that could inform county health departments and the Pennsylvania Department of Health on policy and planning around children's issues during a disaster.
- Create an ad hoc taskforce for electronic health record (EHR) integration into public health activities.

Bidirectional Communication

- *Public Health:* Expand the Health Alert Network; use conference calls and websites to bring pediatric practices better situational awareness during disasters; define data needs (e.g., disease surveillance, mental health outcomes, long-term care outcomes); create a child health desk at the Emergency Operations Center.
- *Pediatricians:* Participate in the Health Alert Network and other communication modalities, and provide feedback.
- *Pennsylvania Chapter of the American Academy of Pediatrics (PA AAP):* Coordinate conference calls and webinars; serve as a communications hub; and convey providers needs to public health.

Communication Between Practices and the Public

- *Public Health:* Integrate practice communication with the public into disaster communication plans; provide early situational awareness, guidance, and support to practices.
- *Pediatricians:* Build capacity through patient portals, phone lines, text messages, social media, websites, and EHRs.
- *PA AAP:* Provide technical assistance and develop a toolkit.

Children with Special Health Care Needs

- *Public Health:* Understand health risks, provide information to pediatricians, coordinate with other public safety agencies, develop new plans and procedures.
- *Pediatricians:* Promote personal preparedness (e.g., evacuation, backup plans, generators, what to bring to a shelter), coordinated care, and the patient-centered medical home model.
- *PA AAP:* Facilitate planning, technical assistance, share guidance and best practices, training.

SOURCE: Chernak presentation, June 10, 2013.

With regard to the creation of the recommended Child Health Advisory Council for Disasters, Chernak noted that the state has agreed to instead create a working group that will inform the state with respect to pediatric issues. Other initiatives will involve planning with schools and child care programs, participation in regional health care coalitions, and practice-based projects such as exercises with local and state agencies.

Chernak cited technology (e.g., EHRs, communications platforms) as one of the major challenges moving forward, and resources are a perpetual challenge. She also highlighted the cultural dissonance between the public health and personal health care systems, and intercounty and interstate differences in priorities as challenges to progress.

In conclusion, Chernak said that a systems-based approach to thinking about public health and health care services is critical. It is important to understand what various partners do relative to each other, and not just prepare individual entities in isolation. Pediatricians play a unique role in the health of children and families, and in support of schools and child care programs and other community institutions. Engaging community medical practices is essential in efforts to prepare communities and build community resilience. A participant added that pediatricians also need to be inculcated into incident command and operations so that children are not forgotten during the implementation.

All panelists discussed further how to get health care systems engaged in preparedness issues. They expressed the importance of taking advantage of that moment in time when people are feeling the impact of lack of preparedness, especially as it affects practice and has financial consequences. For example, after a major storm where practices lose power for 3 to 4 days, providers recognize that they might lose their records, lose $60,000 worth of vaccines, or may not be able to communicate with patients, Chernak said. Hunt added that a motivating force for a health care delivery system is the realization that they need to get back to normal business operations as soon as possible. They lose millions of dollars per day by canceling elective surgeries, for example. Frost and Blake agreed, and Frost said that they take advantage of every unfortunate situation in order to point out the pediatric component to it. She reiterated the value of telling a compelling story, noting that the statewide bed capacity analysis she did for California was instrumental in bringing people to the table. Chernak noted that because drawing providers in to preparedness training before an event is so challenging,

AAP is also building capacity to conduct webinars immediately after disasters, lining up subject-matter experts so that they can provide key information to 1,000 or more pediatricians rapidly.

EVIDENCE-INFORMED GUIDELINES FOR CHILD-FOCUSED PANDEMIC PLANNING AND RESPONSE

Ginny Sprang, executive director of the Center on Trauma and Children at the University of Kentucky, described the development of evidence-informed disaster guidelines intended to optimize preparedness and response for pediatric populations, and prevent adverse unintended consequences (e.g., panic, noncompliance, poor behavioral health outcomes). Citing the work of noted sociologist Robert Merton, Sprang said that well-intended policies and plans inevitably generate unintended consequences that cannot always be anticipated (Merton, 1936). Leaders are under great pressure to act very decisively in situations that, by their nature, are unique and transactional. Error is an unavoidable component of all social action. Strategies generally address proximal outcomes and it is difficult to anticipate the undesired impacts of more distal outcomes.

The research for the project "Evidence-Informed Guidelines for Child-Focused Pandemic Planning and Response" was done at the University of Kentucky in partnership with the University of Louisville, with funding from the Department of Homeland Security through the Kentucky Critical Infrastructure Program.[2] Based on a systematic literature review, Sprang and colleagues developed a toolkit of mixed-method measures (e.g., interview guides, surveys, focus groups, guides, content analysis templates) to collect information from key stakeholders on the gaps and vulnerabilities in systems. Data were collected from diverse stakeholders in six U.S. cities; Mexico City and Juarez, Mexico; and Toronto, Canada (data collection occurred coincidentally as the 2009 H1N1 pandemic influenza was emerging). The findings were used to draft preliminary guidelines which were field tested at the national and

---

[2]Sprang referred participants to the full report, available at http://www.uky.edu/CTAC/sites/www.uky.edu.CTAC/files/NIHS_Del_5i_online_copy_revised__FINAL.pdf (accessed September 9, 2013).

local levels. The final recommendations were then formulated and disseminated as a 3-hour Web-based training program.[3]

Using the University of California, Los Angeles, Post-traumatic Stress Disorder Reaction Index (PTSD-RI), Sprang and colleagues identified a relationship between a disease containment experience and traumatic stress symptoms. Based on the qualitative responses during focus groups, Sprang said that there is something about the disease containment experience that is stigmatizing and stressful in a way that just having H1N1 or severe acute respiratory syndrome (SARS) is not. Parents and children who had no isolation or quarantine experience during either the SARS or H1N1 outbreaks had a mean PTSD-RI score of 5.3, while those who had an isolation or quarantine experience had a mean score of about 22. The anxiety and panic identified in those affected by a health-related disaster triage is complex, and triage, assessment, and intervention strategies are not tailored to these needs. For example, pediatric behavioral health screening was not routine; screening that was done was not evidence-based and not consistent; and screening of family members was rare. Screening also occurred more often in hospital settings versus community settings, and screening for traumatic stress reaction was limited. The relationship between pandemic containment and PTSD symptoms is significant, Sprang explained. About 33 percent of the children who experienced quarantine in isolation met the criteria for posttraumatic stress disorder based on parent reports, as did 25 percent of parents based on their own self-reports. Sprang also highlighted the correlation between parent and child symptoms; about 86 percent of the parents who met the clinical cutoff score for PTSD had children who also met the cutoff. Of those parents who did not meet the cutoff, only about 14 percent of their children met the cutoff. (Sprang acknowledged the potential for contamination of parental perception in the reporting of child symptoms, but noted that young children take behavioral cues from their parents.)

These findings suggest that individual parents and children who experience quarantine or isolation may need behavioral health and other support services to prevent or mitigate these traumatic effects. Sprang and colleagues recommended routine peri- and post-pandemic behavioral health assessment, including trauma screening, for parents and youth who experience isolation or quarantine. Positive identification of PTSD

---

[3]The Web-based training program is available at http://www.cecentral.com/node/433 (accessed September 9, 2013).

in individuals indicates the need for an automatic assessment for the presence of behavioral health disorders in those individuals' family members.

Vulnerabilities

Shifting from parent and child isolation issues to hospital emergency planning, Sprang highlighted several areas of vulnerability identified by the research. For example, hospitals reported that neonatal intensive care units (NICUs) and pediatric intensive care units (PICUs) (which require highly specialized skillsets) were especially vulnerable to staff shortages, even under mild pandemic conditions. Personnel backup plans were often insufficient as available personnel did not have the specialized expertise. To address this, Sprang and colleagues recommended cross-training for areas of potential shortage and three-deep coverage plans.

Prolonged closure of schools creates other vulnerabilities, especially for children who rely on subsidized lunch programs. Sprang noted that few districts were aware of the Pandemic Supplemental Nutrition Assistance Program (P-SNAP),[4] and most did not have a plan for food distributions if schools were closed 5 days or longer. In this regard, the recommendations call for further training and education about P-SNAP and development of a food distribution plan to accommodate worker illness or unavailability.

Need for State and Local Pediatric Module

In terms of the state pandemic preparedness and response plans, there was an underlying assumption in the plans that there would be tight coordination across systems, but Sprang noted that frequent staff turnover often results in the exit of responders with pediatric expertise. At the local level, there was an absence of key stakeholders in planning,

[4]"Section 746 of Public Law 111-80, the Agriculture, Rural Development, Food and Drug Administration, and Related Agencies Appropriations Act, 2010 (signed October 21, 2009) authorizes the Secretary of Agriculture to approve State SNAP agency plans to provide SNAP benefits to households including children certified as eligible to receive free or reduced price school lunches who are enrolled in a school or school district that will be or has been closed for at least 5 consecutive days due to a pandemic emergency." See http://www.fns.usda.gov/sites/default/files/SP_05_SFSP_03-2010_os.pdf (accessed September 9, 2013).

due again in some cases to staff turnover. Activities focused on building resilient response systems occurred generally just before and during a pandemic event, with limited attention between events. In addition, most plans were adult-focused, but did not address the needs of parents. Although 36 percent of the state plans acknowledge the need for family-level disaster planning, there was little focus on operations or guidance regarding what the essential elements of a plan might be. Only 20 percent of the plans contained any guidelines regarding the design, focus, or implementation of behavioral health triage for pediatric populations.

In response, Sprang and colleagues in June 2011 highlighted the need for all state and local pandemic preparedness and response plans to include a module on pediatric health and behavioral health. Behavioral health professionals should be included in the development of these modules. Recommended elements of such pediatric-focused behavioral health module include

- Clearly defined organizational structure for pediatric response coordination.
- Sample risk messaging targeted to children and families.
- Psychoeducational materials that are developmentally informed.
- Alternative behavioral health service delivery options.
- Listing of pediatric-focused, community-based resources to address psychosocial needs.
- Strategies for just-in-time training.
- Continuum of evidence-informed, pediatric-focused interventions.
- Criteria for evidence-informed, protocol-driven behavioral health response.
- Pediatric-specific ethical and legal guidance.

DEVELOPMENT OF A STATE PEDIATRIC AND NEONATAL SURGE ANNEX

Evelyn Lyons, Emergency Medical Services for Children Manager for the Illinois Department of Public Health, detailed her state's development of a pediatric and neonatal surge annex, an appendix to the state medical disaster plan. The annex, developed with funding from the Hospital Preparedness Program cooperative agreements, provides guidance to hospitals and other health care personnel in the event of a large surge of pediatric or neonatal patients.

Illinois is the fifth most populated state in the country, with a total population of 12.8 million, including 2.7 million children (age 15 years and younger). The state has 200 hospitals, 190 of which have emergency departments. Pediatric resources for Illinois children include 15 PICUs and 24 NICUs, 3 of which are actually located in Saint Louis, Missouri, just over the southwest border of the state. Similar to what Frost observed in California, Lyons said that there was a decrease of about 400 licensed pediatric hospital beds within Illinois between 2007 and 2010 (dropping from 2,159 to 1,722). This is particularly concerning in the central and southern part of Illinois, she said, where there are already limited pediatric resources.

Following the release of the National Commission on Children and Disasters report in 2010, Illinois convened a stakeholder group to develop a statewide pediatric and neonatal strategic plan addressing medical surge capabilities and health care system preparedness for at-risk populations. Four workgroups were charged with addressing communication, the decision-making process, system decompression, and standards of care. Lyons provided examples of tools developed by each of the working groups.[5] The communications workgroup developed a Pediatric and Neonatal Event Notification Form, a flow chart that guides users through the activation of the surge annex and the notification of key stakeholders and partners.

The decision-making process workgroup developed an algorithm to guide requests for pediatric medical resources. The algorithm includes consultation with pediatric care medical specialists. These are physicians and nurses who are not onsite, but who provide consultation and guidance at the state level in the event of a surge of pediatric patients. The working group defined the roles, responsibilities, and educational requirements of these experts, and developed just-in-time training that these consultants could utilize during an event.

The system decompression workgroup was responsible for developing a method to decompress tertiary care centers. In the event of a large pediatric surge, pediatric tertiary care centers need to be reserved for more critically ill and injured children, and children with conditions that are less urgent may be able to be moved to community hospitals. Hospitals were asked to self-select from the following categories to describe themselves:

---

[5]All tools referenced can be found in the "Illinois Department of Public Health ESF-8 Plan, Pediatric and Neonatal Surge Annex Attachments" as of September 2013.

- Category one, pediatric tertiary care centers with PICUs and NICUs that care for any level of patient;
- Category two, community hospitals with some pediatric services for children ages 0 to 12 years (including emergency departments approved for pediatric level);
- Category three, community hospitals with no pediatric or neonatal capabilities that could accept pediatric patients ages 12 years and older; and
- Category four, community hospitals with nurseries that can manage pediatric patients ages 0 to 1 year old.

Lyons noted that the system is based on the decompression model developed by Frost for California, showing the benefit of collaboration between states.

Finally, the standards of care workgroup developed a method to track pediatric patients and aid in the reunification of children with their families. They also designed an objective system to triage pediatric patients to tertiary care centers, and a mechanism for communicating patient information between hospitals and with the pediatric care medical specialist. In addition the workgroup developed a series of patient care guidelines for hospitals less familiar with pediatric patients, advising them on care for the first 96 hours after an event, or until they are able to route the children to a higher level of care or to specialty care as needed. Care guidelines cover, for example, burn care, newborn care, premature newborns, radiation, shocks, and other potential pediatric scenarios.

Stakeholders were key to the whole process, Lyons asserted. The process was also advanced by adapting other state resources, such as the Contra Costa County Decompression Model and New York's hospital guidelines for pediatric preparedness. The pediatric annex also serves as a framework for other at-risk populations such as burn surge. There is still work to be done, however. The next steps, Lyons said, emphasizing the theme of drills, are to exercise and test the annex, and modify as needed, and to work with regional health care coalitions to integrate these pediatric concepts into regional planning. Coordination of resources, patient tracking, and liability issues also need to be addressed.

Considerations for children's needs can come from various sectors and organizations. Speakers in this session noted that adapting resources from other states and jurisdictions like Illinois can be helpful if resources are strained and beginning a brand new plan is not feasible. Also, including research and information gathered from focus groups can help to ensure additions to plans have the correct personnel identified and the right inclusions. Finally, Anderson reiterated, breaking down silos and fostering relationships among public health, pediatric providers, and researchers can lead to better response when needed.

5

Financing Health Care for Children in Emergencies

Highlights of Points Made by Individual Speakers

- Investments in improved day-to-day operations for children can also provide extraordinary benefits for emergency preparedness (dual use).
- Private practice pediatricians already do many of the activities needed in a disaster on a daily basis, yet they are essentially left out of all phases of disaster preparedness, response, and recovery.
- Children are covered by many forms of private and public insurance and there is no single database of children's health information, making data collection and analysis challenging.
- State-to-state differences in coverage levels and laws make it challenging to develop broad solutions to payment for children's health services. In addition, many children cross state lines for care.
- Private insurers can be key partners in disaster preparedness and response in many ways, from waiving copays to rebuilding lost patient health records or tracking patient transport from claims data to providing medically trained volunteers and building space.
- Reimbursement pays for intervention. Any time spent away from seeing patients is lost revenue for a private practitioner.
- As for-profit entities, private practice providers are not eligible for grant money from the Department of Health and Human Services or for Federal Emergency Management Agency assistance.

In this section of the report, panelists representing a health system, an insurer, a hospital, and community practice offer their perspectives on the challenges of funding preparedness activities and response. Session chair John Wible, formerly with the Alabama Department of Public Health, offered his own recommendations for several activities an advocacy group could undertake in this area. For example, he suggested becoming familiar with the State Medicaid Agency's policy on out-of-state reimbursement, and working with the agency on cooperation and reimbursement for both in-state and out-of-state care. Educating and encouraging providers close to state borders to sign up for both states' Medicaid network was another consideration along with drafting a model state Pediatric Emergency Preparedness Act to present to state legislators. Finally, he said, working with the Centers for Medicare & Medicaid Services (CMS) to help load the Disproportionate Share Hospital formula in favor of hospitals that join a regional disaster compact would be a good effort that could benefit from advocacy. The rest of this section gives varying financial perspectives of preparedness financing related to children, including the federal level, private insurer, hospital association, and private practice provider. Their considerations and suggestions can help to understand the biggest challenges in this area and where the opportunities for improvement lie.

HEALTH CARE SYSTEM POLICY

Emergency preparedness is built on the strength of everyday health care systems, and the financial stability and sustainability of private-sector health care delivery systems is an essential component of the health security of the nation, said Gregg Margolis, director of the Division of Health System Policy at the Office of the Assistant Secretary for Preparedness and Response. More than 90 percent of the health care delivered in the United States, both routine and during disasters and public health emergencies, is delivered in the private sector.

Health care financing is complex, Margolis said, and there are disparities in the financial stability of various health systems in the United States. Some health care systems report revenue minus expenses of hundreds of millions of dollars per year. Other health care systems, often those that serve vulnerable populations, are much less financially stable. Disasters disproportionately affect vulnerable populations, and pediatric populations in particular, and Margolis emphasized the need to address the financial stability of safety net providers that will be further stressed during public health emergencies and disasters.

Disasters affect the entire health care system. Although there is much discussion about emergency care or trauma care systems, a public health emergency also impacts the primary care system, long-term care, nursing homes, behavioral health, ambulatory care, and specialty care. There are considerable threats or costs to a health care system during a disaster, for example, unanticipated expenses, business interruption, lost revenue, lost workforce, increased proportion of uncompensated care, and liability. However, disasters are low-frequency events, and low-financial-return types of investments. It can be very difficult to convince health care administrators to invest their limited resources in disaster preparedness when they are inundated by other institutional priorities that have a high probability of being used and will generate high returns on investment (e.g., imaging technologies, laboratory services).

One approach to paying for preparedness is through grant funding. Another way to fund preparedness is as part of the cost of doing business. In a fee-for-service environment, where volume generates revenue through reimbursement, a small fraction of every dollar generated goes toward paying for preparedness. However, as noted above, many programs compete for a portion of this small fraction. Margolis suggested that payment/reimbursement for care during disasters (especially emergency or trauma services) could create a revenue source. But disasters disproportionately affect vulnerable populations, which are disproportionately self-pay or Medicaid patients.

Shifting the Mindset

The challenge, Margolis said, is shifting the financial mindset from emergency preparedness as an investment, to emergency preparedness as insurance. How do we make emergency preparedness an integral part of the entire U.S. health care system, beyond the emergency care system, critical care, and emergency medical services? Margolis suggested that a successful business case for emergency preparedness involves decreasing the cost and increasing the value of preparedness. As the health care system evolves from a fee-for-service, volume-based reimbursement system, to a value-based reimbursement system, how do we ensure that preparedness is part of the value equation? One mechanism to increase value is to focus on activities that build from and leverage day-to-day functions to strengthen preparedness and response. As an example, Margolis pointed to how investments in health information technology infrastructure have improved day-to-day operations but have also provided extraordinary benefits for emergency preparedness. To decrease the cost of emergency preparedness on individual facilities, Margolis called for increased collaboration, coalition building, and new partnerships, so that the burden is shared by all of the institutions when a disaster or public health emergency affects a community. Margolis also described a model of "coopetition" that has been very successful in the airline industry. In this model, organizations that normally compete against each other for market share of their services agree to cooperate in certain defined spaces for the advancement of all. In health care, emergency preparedness could be one such area for coopetition.

The task moving forward, Margolis reiterated, is to think not only about how to build a financially sustainable health care system, but how to ensure that emergency preparedness is an integral part of the entire evolving health care system.

PRIVATE INSURERS

Robert Smith, senior medical director for the central region of United Healthcare Clinical Services, began by clarifying that UnitedHealth Group is both an insurer, through its UnitedHealthcare division, and a health and wellness company, through its Optum division. Together, these two divisions employ more than 133,000 staff, including 27,000 physicians, nurses, and other clinical practitioners, and 12,000 technologists. United manages more than $300 billion in health care annually, and invests more than $2 billion in technology and new development. United delivers health care through the management of medical groups and hospice, and through direct clinical, pharmacy, and health financial services. Overall, United serves 83 million consumers, 777,000 care providers, and 250,000 plan sponsors.

Smith listed some of the many ways that health care for a child is paid for. Employer-based insurance programs can be fully insured plans with coverage provided by a major insurer (e.g., UnitedHealthcare, Anthem, Cigna) or they can be self-funded plans where the employer hires a firm to manage the transactions for them (as is done by the federal government). Smith added that self-insured employers have a lot of control over the process. Other examples include individual policies, self-paid policies, Medicaid, state health insurance programs, military health care, the Indian Health Service, and programs for children with special needs or those under the care of the state (e.g., foster children, those in the juvenile justice system).

The system of payment is complex, which makes it difficult to evaluate data from across the nation regarding coverage. Smith used data from the Kaiser Family Foundation regarding coverage of children ages 0 to 18 to highlight some of the disparities in coverage. In Connecticut, Massachusetts, Minnesota, and Utah, for example, 64 percent of children are covered by employer-based programs, and in New Hampshire is it 68 percent. In Arkansas, Louisiana, and New Mexico, it is 38 percent or less.

Differences in coverage levels and laws from state to state make it challenging to develop broad solutions to payment for children's health services. In addition, many children cross state lines for care. Large numbers of children are covered by private plans, and it can be difficult to coordinate between carriers, and difficult to identify the responsible parties. Additional challenges to payment for children's health services listed by Smith include the lack of population-based health system responses, and lack of accountable organizations for care and financing. He added that the effectiveness and adequacy of public–private partnerships is highly variable, and the needs and expectations exceed the ability to respond of any single organization.

Smith called out several key differences between private and public insurance that are important in disasters. In private insurance, the eligibility of a child for payment of care depends on the employment of parents. In the public sector payment is independent of parental employment. Importantly, some items (e.g., dental needs, therapy, private duty nursing) are quite commonly paid for by public coverage, but are subject to restrictions and limits, or not covered at all by private insurance. In a disaster, the majority of children may be covered by employer or individual insurance; however, they may become separated from their parents. These children are not likely to have identification or a health insurance card in their pocket, and may not be able to provide accurate health histories. Their clinical records are likely with private practitioners and may be inaccessible or destroyed, and as such, immediate specialized care may not be available to them.

Roles of Insurance Providers in Disasters

As an insurer, Smith said that a company like UnitedHealth Group has a variety of resilience and response roles, including providing for the safety of its employees. From a business perspective, the company strives to minimize service disruptions, preserve customer information and organizational assets (including people, process, technology, and information), and continue to comply with laws and regulations regarding continuity of operations. The UnitedHealth Group business continuity plans focus on critical business functions and planning for the worst-case scenario so that the organization can react quickly and efficiently, even in the face of loss of its own critical systems, resources, or facilities.

Because private insurers control a significant portion of health care dollars as the fiduciary representatives of employers of parents, they can have significant involvement in disaster preparedness and response. For example, insurers can waive the copay for prescriptions refill for medications lost in the disaster. They can cover visits to out-of-network providers at the higher in-network payment levels. If provider records are destroyed or the provider cannot be found, Smith said that United-Healthcare can compile a profile of a given child's medical situation by using information from health claims such as diagnoses and prescriptions. Claims data can also be used to track patient transport and reunite families. As a large employer and business, insurers have medical staff who can volunteer, and facilities that can serve as shelters or auxiliary medical sites. Smith stressed the importance of public–private partnership and urged planners to include insurers in preparedness discussions.

HOSPITAL ASSOCIATION

The mission of the Children's Hospital Association is to advance children's health through the quality, cost, and delivery of care in association with the 225 member hospitals, said Amy Knight, senior vice president of the Children's Hospital Association. Members include freestanding children's hospitals as well as pediatric units within larger hospitals or health systems. Many of the children cared for by the network of children's hospitals have complex medical conditions, and many are children who are covered by Medicaid. These populations are particularly vulnerable in a disaster.

Knight listed the primary activities of the Children's Hospital Association as public policy and advocacy; data, research, and analysis; peer networking and knowledge exchange among members; clinical quality and operational improvements; and purchasing and cost containment initiatives. Knight noted that one of the challenges with regard to data and analysis is that the pediatric population is covered by various forms of private and public insurance and there is no single database of children's health information. Day-to-day issues drive hospital priorities and often trump planning and preparedness activities, Knight explained. Those issues and priorities include, for example, patient safety; Medicaid (and paying for children's care in the face of Medicaid budget cuts); workforce, including subspecialty recruitment and training; value (i.e., competitiveness on quality and cost of care); market strategy; and organizational survival.

Advancing preparedness can be overwhelming for children's hospitals, in large part because they are only part of the system. They are largely focused on acute care (i.e., response) rather than preparedness. Similarly, reimbursement pays for intervention, not for prevention or preparedness. The availability of resources, both internally and externally, is a perpetual challenge, and she concurred with Margolis that capital investment decisions are generally for something that has an immediate return on investment. Population health and accountable care are in nascent stages of development, Knight said, as there are very few children's hospitals, and most children are not treated at children's hospitals.

Knight suggested that one potential driver of change in the way children's hospitals invest in preparedness is their expanding accountability, influence, and control across the care continuum. External incentives and expectations also drive change (e.g., reimbursement, grants, regulations, certifications, standards). Ultimately, current events are major drivers of change and force people to think differently about preparedness.

INDEPENDENT PRIVATE PRACTICE PROVIDERS

The majority of pediatric care is primary care provided by pediatricians, as well as family practitioners, nurse practitioners, and physician assistants, said Scott Needle, a pediatrician in the Healthcare Network of Southwest Florida (Phillips et al., 2005). There are also cognitive subspecialists and surgical subspecialists who focus on pediatric care. The majority of pediatric care takes place in independent private practices, which Needle said can range from solo practices to "super groups" such as Pediatric Associates in South Florida, which has

180 pediatricians at 25 sites. Pediatric care also takes place in health care systems, hospital-owned practices, and federally qualified health centers.

Medicaid is the single largest payer of children's health care, covering 39 percent of the children in the United States. Children in families who do not qualify for Medicaid, but still have limited income, may be covered by the State Children's Health Insurance Program (SCHIP). Many children are covered in some fashion by private insurers, and some are self-paying. Children are not covered by Medicare, Needle reminded participants. This is an important point because Medicare is a federal government program with uniform coverage across the country, while Medicaid, although funded in part by the federal government, is run by the states and coverage can vary. After Hurricane Katrina, for example, Medicare incentive payments were made available for some of the affected providers and institutions. Any kind of comparable proactive change to Medicaid is much more difficult to effect because four agencies are involved in the decisions (CMS, Congress, the state legislature, and the state Medicaid authority).

Medicaid is generally one of the lowest-paying payers for most pediatric providers, Needle said. The current payment system is fee-for-service, which means the pediatrician is paid for face-to-face encounters with the patients. Any time spent away from seeing patients (such as giving a talk at an Institute of Medicine workshop, or spending time on preparedness) is lost revenue. In addition, payments are generally preset and inflexible and there is no ability to recoup losses suffered by a practice during a disaster. There are also many administrative and regulatory burdens which can be particularly challenging for small practices with limited administrative staff.

Challenges in Engaging Providers

Needle continued by noting that outside agencies attempting to engage pediatricians in preparedness face several challenges. First, pediatric providers are fragmented, diverse, and independent. There is no central agency or authority through which on can reach out to all providers. For example, although The Joint Commission does have outpatient certification, the average pediatrician has no incentive or reason to participate. Office-based providers are also for-profit entities, and Needle explained that they are not eligible for grant money from the Department of Health and Human Services or other agencies unless there is a specific provision. In addition, the Stafford Act does not allow for Federal Emergency Management Agency assistance directly to for-profit businesses in a disaster. The net result is that office-based providers are essentially left out of all phases of disaster preparedness, response, and recovery.

This is a significant concern because providers have a significant role in the community. For the majority of people, an office-based provider is their first point of contact with the health care system. Pediatricians hope to see 100 percent of their patients in the office at least once every year for annual well care, or routine acute or chronic care. Care provided in the office can often prevent someone from having to go to the emergency room, Needle said. In addition to providing care that can lead to overall health system cost savings, providers also have a positive economic impact on their communities. Needle cited an American Medical Association (AMA) study that found that, on average, each individual office-based physician generates about $100,000 in state and local tax revenue each year (AMA, 2011). In aggregate, office-based physicians are a tremendous part of local and state economies in the United States. In 46 out of 50 states, for example, physician practices across all specialties paid out more in employee wages and benefits than the hospital systems in the same states. In some states, physicians pay out more in employee wages and benefits than hospitals, universities, home health care agencies, nursing homes, and legal facilities combined in the same states.

As discussed earlier by Chernak (see Chapter 3), physicians also have a significant role to play in a disaster. Many of the activities necessary in response to a disaster are already done every day by the office-based pediatrician (e.g., communication, public health surveillance, vaccines, longitudinal care, mental and behavior health). This is dual use capacity waiting to be tapped, he said. Needle added that office-based providers are key partners in a disaster for the management of children with special health care needs.

Opportunities for Preparedness

Involving private practice pediatricians in preparedness, response, and recovery will require financial and material assistance. Needle suggested that there are some current opportunities that can be leveraged for preparedness. For example, the meaningful use standards for electronic health records (EHRs) allows providers to earn incentive payments, and increases the functionality of their EHR systems. The Affordable Care Act does not address preparedness per se, but the Medicaid parity to Medicare provision does allow for higher Medicaid payment rates, which could create more possibilities for preparedness. The patient-centered medical home model of care fulfills many of the criteria for disaster-based capabilities. Finally, accountable care organizations are moving health care toward a value-based continuum of care, which also means a shift toward population-based or community pediatric care, creating the potential to help many more children, Needle said. It also provides the opportunities for collaboration, networking, and data collection.

Other opportunities include community coalitions, and networks to share resources and create economies of scale. Needle also suggested recovery memoranda of understanding or contracts that could pass on Stafford Act disaster recovery funds to office-based practices, perhaps similar to how for-profit debris removal services are contracted by the state for disaster services.

Bruce Clements of the Texas Department of State Health Services raised an additional financial issue for private providers. He relayed the concerns of a private provider following Hurricane Katrina who felt that the disaster clinics were putting the provider out of business. States are good at quickly deploying resources when needed, but deciding when is the right time to demobilize medical assets post-disaster is a very difficult decision, Clements said. It is a delicate balance between supporting the community and threatening the current infrastructure. Needle concurred noting that the free clinics were often the only source of care in the first few days to weeks after Hurricane Katrina. But as time went on, patients wondered why they should pay a $20 copay at their providers office when they can go to the free clinic instead. Experience from Haiti and other disasters shows that staying too long can set up this care conflict and actually undermine the self-sufficiency of the local health care system. Needle suggested the need for a regional health care coordinator: someone who could coordinate and assess the health care situation from the integrated system as a whole, and better define current needs. Moving forward, coordinating the needs of children through private practice providers, private insurers, hospitals, and federal-level policy makers could help to alleviate the disjointed framework that currently plagues reimbursement and finance for children's care after disasters.

6

Broadening Stakeholders Invested in Children

Highlights of Points Made by Individual Speakers

- Availability of child care is a critical component of recovery; it allows parents to attend to their business, such as applying for aid and other recovery activities.
- The spiritual and religious needs of faith communities are generally lacking in mass care and mass fatality planning, which can have detrimental effects on children. Including spiritual and religious groups in planning can also build a better communication network to families.
- Greater religious literacy and competency is needed in emergency management and public health; specific consideration should be placed on the needs of children in disasters and the effects of emotional and spiritual trauma.
- Youth who are trained in preparedness become more resilient and are highly effective messengers, engaging their peers, parents, and other adults.

Typically, in planning stages, public health and emergency planners will include partners within their sectors or other leaders of government who are involved or directly related to formulating a successful response. However, with certain sections of the population, children especially, including nontraditional community partners can allow for better and more comprehensive planning and response. In this chapter, some examples of nontraditional partners are explored, from child care providers to those who serve special populations of children such as individuals with disabilities, faith communities, and engaged youth. A theme mentioned in earlier chapters—bringing together a diverse set of stakeholders when adding children and family needs to emergency plans—can assist in making the outcomes more realistic and the tactics more viable.

PREPAREDNESS ISSUES FOR CHILD CARE

Linda Smith, Deputy Assistant Secretary and Inter-Departmental Liaison for Early Childhood Development at the Administration for Children and Families (ACF), provided an overview of child care in the United States and highlighted some of the preparedness issues for child care at the federal, local, and provider levels. Painting a picture of child care providers across the country, Smith explained that there are about 2.1 million child care workers in the United States, with an annual turnover rate of about 30 percent. Average salary for a child care worker is $21,000 per year, which Smith pointed out is poverty level for a family of three. Child care workers are 98 percent female, many have only a high school education or less, and half are eligible for public assistance. Roughly 12 million children in the United States aged 5 years old and younger are in child care. One million children are in centers, about 250,000 are in family home-based child care, and the rest are in some form of in-home or relative care. Child care takes place in neighborhoods, strip malls, and churches. It is for-profit and nonprofit. Child care is not a universal system, Smith stressed.

Smith described several examples of child care–related activities at the federal level. For example, the Federal Emergency Management Agency (FEMA) released a recovery fact sheet on public assistance for child care services to help the public to understand what FEMA can and cannot do with regard to child care in the aftermath of a disaster.[1] FEMA and ACF also sent a joint letter to state governors asking them to include child care in their state emergency plans.[2] When child care is not included in the plans, the providers are not eligible for FEMA reimbursement, making recovery even more difficult.

At the local level, it is important for first responders to know where child care is taking place in their communities. To help with this, the federal government has funded some projects to map child care in communities, Smith noted. It is also important to back up the local data

---

[1] See http://www.acf.hhs.gov/sites/default/files/occ/fema_public_assistance_for_child_care_services.pdf (accessed October 28, 2013).

[2] The FEMA and ACF letter can be found at http://www.acf.hhs.gov/programs/occ/resource/acf-and-fema-joint-letter-to-state-governors (accessed October 28, 2013).

regarding children in child care. A child care provider may have parents in their database, and a city may have child care providers in a database, but this needs to be backed up and remotely available so that it is accessible when needed.

Finally, at the provider level, Smith reiterated, preparedness is "more than a fire drill." Providers need assistance in developing plans and Smith noted several specific needs, listed below:

- A call-in system: Child care providers can contact a central location to report their status during a disaster.
- Age-specific materials: These are currently lacking and could be useful for providers when working with young children who have been traumatized.
- Up-to-date information from parents (e.g., how to reach them in an emergency, medications the child may need to have if evacuated).
- Funding for preparedness activities: Given the limited income of a child care provider, this is especially needed.

Although needs and gaps exist, child care remains a critical component of response and recovery. Parents need to clean up, pick up, move or rebuild, stand in lines for assistance, and return to work. At the same time, child care providers are also trying to rebuild their home or business. Providers themselves are part of the impacted community and are also traumatized. Providers are not automatically trained to deal with traumatized children. Facilities may be damaged and closed, and if a facility is closed for 2 or 3 months, it may go out of business. In closing, Smith referred participants to emergency standards for child care developed by Save the Children and the National Association of Child Care Resource and Referral Agencies (now Child Care Aware).[3]

COMMUNITY ENGAGEMENT

Among many other organizations, FEMA has recently embraced and encouraged a "whole community" approach when it comes to emergency planning and response and recovery. Parallel with that concept, a continuous theme throughout the workshop was that the involved

---

[3]Available at http://www.naccrra.org/sites/default/files/publications/naccrra_publications/2012/protectingchildreninchildcareemergencies.pdf (accessed September 9, 2013).

stakeholders in planning discussions need to be broadened past that of just pediatricians and child-focused hospital coalitions. Stakeholders should include organizations and representatives across all sectors that work or interact with children, including schools, youth groups, religious organizations, and others. This section brings together nontraditional partners who represent community groups that can be leveraged for better community engagement and buy-in and improved risk communication and message dissemination.

Planning for the Needs of People with Disabilities

Easter Seals is a social service organization focused on providing services and support to people with disabilities. Patricia Wright, national director of autism services at Easter Seals, said that in 2012, the organization provided direct service to 1.6 million people with disabilities in the United States, more than half of whom were children.

Wright listed 13 categories of disability: specific learning disabilities, speech or language impairments, intellectual disability, emotional disturbance, hearing impairments, orthopedic impairments, other health impairments, visual impairments, multiple disabilities, deaf-blindness, autism, traumatic brain injury, and developmental delay. Wright noted that the needs of those with physical disabilities or orthopedic impairments are often raised in preparedness planning discussions, but learning, intellectual, emotional, and speech and language disabilities are also prominent in society. People with disabilities have unique needs; for example, children with autism are subject to wandering. Many children with intellectual disabilities also have parents with intellectual disabilities who will need services and support.

Wright listed several resources available specifically for people with disabilities. The Rehabilitation Engineering Research Center (RERC) has developed specific tools for use with individuals who have complex communication needs, including, for example, a universal communication access board that uses pictograms and pictures for communication.[4] The universal design of such devices makes them useful not only for communication with people who are nonverbal or have low literacy rates, but also with people who speak other languages.

[4]RERC resources available at http://aac-rerc.psu.edu/index.php/pages/show/id/4 (accessed September 9, 2013).

Another tool is a "go bag" filled with the unique items a person with a disability might need to take with them in an emergency (e.g., a communication board, medicines and supplies, food, clothing). Relaxation techniques are also useful for people with disabilities. The Oregon Health Science University (OHSU) and the Green Mountain Emergency Preparedness Project at the University of Vermont also have emergency preparedness toolkits for people with disabilities.[5]

Wright urged state and local planners to include people with disabilities or their representatives in planning groups. Organizations with disability expertise to share include, for example, the University Centers for Excellence in Developmental Disabilities, Family Voices, Community Council on Developmental Disabilities, and Centers for Independent Living.

Engaging Faith Communities

The American religious landscape is a mosaic, as diverse as the population, said Peter Gudaitis, chief response officer for New York Disaster Interfaith Services and president of the National Disaster Interfaiths Network. About 90 percent of Americans say they are religious or spiritual, and 43 percent of Americans say that they attend worship services regularly at approximately 345,000 U.S. houses of worship. The United States is the most Christian country in the world. Eighty percent of Americans self-identify as Christian, although the percentage is decreasing due to demographic shifts in the population. Today, for example, there are more Muslims in the United States than there are Episcopalians and Presbyterians. Americans are connecting with their religious institutions as places of learning and communication, and Gudaitis added that activities such as religious education, Bible study, and youth groups probably account for the most significant percentage of institutional relationships outside of schools.

Faith communities have historically responded to disasters and human suffering. There is growing interest from government for greater faith community engagement, and a growing interest from and need for faith communities to work with government on disasters. There are

[5]The OHSU toolkit is available at http://www.ohsu.edu/xd/research/centers-institutes/institute-on-development-and-disability/public-health-programs/oodh-emergency-preparedness.cfm; University of Vermont toolkit available at http://www.uvm.edu/~cdci/gmep (accessed September 9, 2013).

significant gaps between these two entities, compounded by what Gudaitis described as an "extraordinary lack of religious literacy and competency." Religious competency, Gudaitis explained, is knowing how to navigate and engage each faith community (and individual adherents) competently and respectfully, as a trusted, knowledgeable, and effective partner. Religious literacy is having a basic understanding of the history, sacred texts, beliefs, and rituals (including diet, clothing) of multiple faith traditions, and the ability to understand the intersection of religions and social, political, and cultural life. The spiritual and religious needs of the faith communities are generally lacking in mass care and mass fatality planning, Gudaitis said. If a Muslim family entered a shelter, for example, would the staff know that the men and women may want to shelter separately, what Halal food is, and whether or not Kosher food would be acceptable instead? Even if the sleeping areas of the shelter were separated by gender, it may still be unacceptable for the women and men to have to walk past each other to the bathrooms.

Helping to Improve Planning

Gudaitis drew from the objectives and recommendations of a project on faith communities and disasters that he has worked on with the Center for Religion and Civic Culture at the University of Southern California (funded by the California Emergency Management Agency). To improve disaster planning for children, he said, we need greater religious literacy and competency in emergency management and public health; competent government outreach to congregations, faith-based organizations, and religious families; and education for religious leaders on the needs of children in disasters and the effects of emotional and spiritual trauma. Disaster planning for children should include faith-based risk communication and public service announcements oriented to the full range of children's ages and/or their caregivers, Gudaitis continued. Religious leaders need information on how to care effectively for children and their congregation, and how to educate parents and their caregivers to care for children in disasters, particularly in minority, immigrant, or non-English-speaking communities. All disaster mental health planning should include the spiritual needs of children and mass care, and mass fatality plans should provide specific direction for the care and disposition of children from religious families.

Gudaitis referred participants to a series of tip sheets developed by the National Disaster Interfaith Network for religious leaders to help them address needs of religious children and families.[6] The back page of each "Be a Ready Congregation" tip sheet also includes information on training resources or education resources. Examples shown were tip sheets addressing children in a disaster and an active shooter in a house of worship. There are also a series of tip sheets for faith community partners which are competency guidelines on issues such as sheltering and mass care of different faith communities with unique dress, diet, or sheltering requirements (e.g., Buddhist, Hindu, Jewish, Muslim, Sikh). Information on how to support children of those faith traditions is included as well. In closing, Gudaitis recommended a text by Stephen Prothero, *Religious Literacy*, to those interested in learning more about religious literacy and competency.

Engaging Youth

Ashley Houston, a high school student and member of FEMA's Youth Preparedness Council, shared her personal experience and perspective on engaging youth in preparedness. Houston became involved in the youth council through a school club called Health Occupations Students of America. Children can play an important role during emergencies and should be a part of all disaster planning, preparedness, response, and recovery efforts, she said. Communities and towns should target teens through schools and community programs because youth who are trained in preparedness become more resilient in actual disasters. Youth are also highly effective messengers who can be used to reach their parents as well as other adults. In addition, engaging youth today will ensure future generations of prepared adults.

The FEMA Youth Preparedness Council gives teenagers an opportunity to voice their opinions, share their experiences, and offer ideas and solutions to help strengthen the nation's resiliency for all types of disasters. The council is comprised of 13 diverse leaders from across the country, ranging in age from 13 to 17, who have demonstrated a willingness to represent the youth perspective on emergency preparedness and to take information back to their communities. Members of the Youth Preparedness Council work on yearlong projects, help to set up

---

[6]More information on the tip sheets for congregations and community partners is available at http://www.n-din.org (accessed September 9, 2013).

regional youth councils, serve as ambassadors of youth preparedness, and provide feedback. Houston described some of her activities, including coordinating and participating in teen Community Emergency Response Team (CERT) demonstrations at local events in her community, and completing the necessary training to become a CERT instructor as well as organizing a course for teens at her school.

Because youth play such an important role in outreach to other audiences, Houston recommended reaching out to them through their school programs. School drills, for example, help prepare children for real emergencies, and they share this information at home with their parents. Most schools also have student resource officers who are law-related counselors and educators in the school who can share information. School clubs are a big part of student's lives and are also a good way to reach students. Houston also offered suggestion on ways to connect with youth outside of schools through youth organizations (e.g., Boy Scouts of America, Girl Scouts of America), church groups, and emergency response programs (e.g., CERT and Teen CERT). Finally, Houston said that Twitter and social media are tools that can be used to connect with and involve youth in preparedness. She added that members of the Youth Preparedness Council have been teaching their advisors how youth use social media tools and how social media can better be used for outreach.

Engaging different parts of the community for their input on planning and assistance in outreach can be a great tool for jurisdictions as they try to promote more awareness and identify gaps in the response and recovery frameworks.

7

Planning for Children and Families During Disaster Response

Highlights of Points Made by Individual Speakers

- Most people with disabilities do not have acute medical needs. Planning to meet the access and functional needs of disaster survivors in general population shelters can help to preserve limited acute care resources for those with a true medical need.
- In the aftermath of a disaster, primary care providers are likely to be the first, and possibly the only, responders to provide mental health services to children.
- Professional staff may be impacted directly themselves and may have some of the same behavioral and mental health needs as those they serve.
- A single disaster event is really part of a cascade of other events in a child's life and results in cumulative impact and stress.
- Stigma related to mental health is a still barrier, even in times of national crisis.
- Temporary child care in shelters and service centers allows parents to attend to business, such as applying for aid and other recovery activities.
- Include older children with disabilities in the process when planning for their evacuation and transportation during an emergency. They know what works for them and what does not.

Planning for the specific needs of children and families in response to disasters, including functional needs, nutritional needs, family reunification, and temporary child care, is extremely important when thinking about community plans. These specific needs are discussed throughout this chapter in addition to real-world experiences that support these needs. Participants also share best practices and potential strategies for response. Examples include regional preparedness, infection prevention, sheltering, tracking, evacuation and transportation of children with disabilities, and novel training techniques.

CHILD AND FAMILY NEEDS DURING MASS CARE AND SHELTERING OPERATIONS

Session chair Kari Tatro, executive vice president of Emergency Management Operations for BCFS Health and Human Services,[1] said that meeting the needs of children in disasters presents a unique set of planning considerations. She gave an overview of logistical requirements and cultural considerations regarding children with medical needs, shelter placement, unaccompanied children, children in state or federal custody, the impact of stress and trauma on children, and neonatal transport and services. When facility plans cannot be implemented, there need to be alternative plans for evacuation, alternate care sites, and field triage sites. To meet the logistical needs of children, planners need to consider the availability of items in shelters such as cribs and crib linens, clothing, food, eating utensils, diapers, pediatric durable medical equipment, and pediatric consumable medical supplies. There are also cultural considerations when sheltering children, especially as they relate to food service. Change in diet (e.g., providing cow's milk to children who have only ever consumed almond milk) can lead to gastrointestinal disorders, vomiting, and diarrhea.

From a medical perspective, there must be access to pediatric medical equipment and medication dosages. Planning considerations also need to include a process for making medical decisions for unaccompanied children. Children will have medical needs that must be addressed with or without their parents present, Tatro said. Similarly, there must be provisions for maintaining a chain of custody for children in state or federal custody for medical decisions.

There are special shelter placement considerations for children with disabilities. Historically, individuals with disabilities have been sent to medical shelters or to medical facilities. Tatro said that children with disabilities should instead be sheltered with their families in general

[1] BCFS is an international health and human services agency that provides all-hazards emergency management, planning, preparedness, and response.

population shelters whenever possible. As such, it is important to ensure adequate planning for children with disabilities in general shelters. If a child has a medical need that requires professional licensed staff oversight, then placement in a medical shelter may be appropriate, but planning should include considerations for keeping the family unit together (instead of splitting the child and one parent away from the rest of the family).

Thinking about mental health, Tatro explained the trauma and stress of disaster and the sheltering experience can impact children differently than adults. New and stressful experiences can include, for example, disease isolation and quarantine, being in a group living situation with thousands of strangers, standing in line to get meals, or trying to find clothing. Educational opportunities, games and recreation, and counseling opportunities, including psychological first aid, can help to alleviate some of the stress and trauma for these children. It is important to draw on partnerships to meet some of those needs, Tatro said. Further mental health considerations for children in emergencies are explored in Chapter 8.

Functional Needs Support Services

The Federal Emergency Management Agency (FEMA) Office of Disability Integration and Coordination was established to provide guidance, tools, methods, and strategies to integrate and coordinate emergency management that is inclusive of children and adults with access and functional needs, in accordance with federal civil rights laws and regulations. Marcie Roth, director of the Office of Disability Integration and Coordination at FEMA, quoted FEMA administrator Craig Fugate, who has stated that "if we wait and plan for people with disabilities after we write the basic plan we fail." In this spirit, FEMA tools and resources are now inclusive of the whole community (rather than addressing some subpopulations in the back of a manual or in a separate annex).

Several federal laws prohibit discrimination in emergency programs on the basis of disability (see Box 7-1). These laws apply to preparation, exercises, notification, evacuation and transportation, sheltering, first aid and medical services, temporary lodging and housing, transition back to the community, clean-up, and other emergency- and disaster-related programs, services, and activities.

BOX 7-1
Federal Laws Prohibiting Discrimination in Emergency Programs on the Basis of Disability

- Rehabilitation Act of 1973
- Americans with Disabilities Act of 1990
- Stafford Act of 1988
- Post Katrina Emergency Management Reform Act of 2006
- Fair Housing Act Amendments of 1988
- Architectural Barriers Act of 1968
- Individuals with Disabilities Education Act of 1975
- Telecommunications Act of 1996
- Twenty-First Century Communications and Video Accessibility Act of 2010

SOURCE: Roth presentation, June 11, 2013.

Roth noted that the term "access and functional needs" is now preferred to the term "special needs," as the latter tends to relegate these issues to annexes, separate documents, and separate plans, she explained, which is the antithesis of inclusion.

In addition to adults and children with physical, mobility, sensory, intellectual, developmental, cognitive, or mental health disabilities, others who may have access and functional needs include older adults, people with chronic or temporary health conditions, women in late stages of pregnancy, as well as those with limited English proficiency or low literacy, no access to transportation, very low income, or who are experiencing homelessness.

It is important to recognize that most people with disabilities do not have acute medical needs and maintain their health, safety and independence in their home and community on a daily basis. Planning to meet the access and functional needs of disaster survivors with and without disabilities in general population shelters can help to keep people out of the acute care setting and preserve limited acute care resources for those who have a true medical need. If given the proper support, people with disabilities can be successfully accommodated in shelters with their family. But providing this support and meeting their access and functional needs requires planning and coordination, and involvement of the whole community. To help guide local governments and communities, Roth referred participants to the FEMA functional needs support services guidance.[2] This tool includes information about planning, finding subject-matter experts, selecting shelter sites, accessible toilets and bathing facilities, personal assistance needs, medical care and equipment, legal obligations, and service animals. Another useful tool Roth highlighted is the FEMA personal assistance services contract.[3] If a disaster situation exceeds a state's ability to meet the needs of people with access and functional needs in general population shelters, FEMA can bring in up to 2,500 personal assistance service providers to assist with both basic and higher-level care.

When communities integrate the access and functional needs of children and adults with and without disabilities in all phases of community-wide emergency management, they strengthen their ability to prepare for, protect against, respond to, recover from, and mitigate all hazards, Roth concluded.

During the discussion, the need for research was discussed and it was noted that there are grant opportunities with the National Institute on Disability and Rehabilitation Research (part of the U.S. Department of Education) focused disability inclusive emergency management practices.

Family Reunification

One of the primary needs of children in the shelter environment is family reunification. Mary Casey-Lockyer, manager of disaster health services at the American Red Cross, discussed several Red Cross programs that help to facilitate family reunification in times of disaster, including the Safe and Well Online Registry, and Patient Connection. Safe and Well is a free, Web-based tool that people can use to let their loved ones, friends, and colleagues know they are safe.[4] Those affected by disasters self-register on the site, and anyone can search the list for friends and family and view the registrants' posted messages. Clients can also update their status on Facebook or Twitter, simply by clicking an

---

[2]The *FEMA Guidance on Planning for Integration of Functional Needs Support Services in General Population Shelters* is available at http://www.fema.gov/pdf/about/odic/fnss_guidance.pdf (accessed September 9, 2013).

[3]Further information on the personal assistance services contract is available at http://www.pascenter.org/publications/item.php?id=1324&focus= (accessed September 9, 2103).

[4]The Red Cross Safe and Well website address is http://www.redcross.org/safeandwell (accessed September 9, 2013).

icon in the Safe and Well registration page. Everyone in their "friends list" will be notified that they registered on the American Red Cross Safe and Well website. This is an integrated response, Casey-Lockyer explained, and Red Cross volunteers also physically locate vulnerable people and conduct welfare checks when a request is initiated by a concerned family member. Safe and Well is available 24 hours per day, every day of the year. In addition to the website, Red Cross also uses paper forms in shelters and at evacuation transition points, and has computer spreadsheets for when Internet connectivity is not available. Roth noted that there are many current initiatives to help with family reunification and patient tracking (e.g., FEMA initiatives, individual state systems, Google Missing Persons, Facebook, Crisis Commons, and others) and the question is how these systems will integrate.

Another Red Cross tool is Patient Connection. The system is currently being used in Chicago and will be implemented statewide in Illinois in the future. The system is triggered if 10 or more people affected by a particular disaster are sent to area hospitals, or by mass-casualty events such as transportation accidents (e.g., mass transit, aviation, traffic emergencies) or building fires and collapses. Patient Connection has also been activated as a precaution before large events such as the Chicago Marathon and the North Atlantic Treaty Organization summit. In these types of situations, disaster victims are frequently transported without notice to their loved ones. Red Cross activates a single hotline for families to call to locate relatives, reducing calls and walk-in traffic to emergency departments. Hospitals send names and descriptions of affected patients to Red Cross, and call agents work to make matches. Hospitals and emergency management can then refer families that call to the Red Cross hotline to locate their loved one. Casey-Lockyer clarified that the Red Cross is exempt from Health Insurance Portability and Accountability Act (HIPAA) privacy rules, and in times of disasters, HIPAA provisions allow hospitals to share information with a recognized response agency such as the Red Cross for reunification purposes.

Casey-Lockyer added that American Red Cross now has a digital disaster operation center, called DigiDOC. The Red Cross can monitor publicly available social media and can push current information back to the public via national communication channels such as Twitter, Facebook, email, and the Red Cross website.

Nutritional Needs

Another primary need of all children in a shelter is nutrition. Casey-Lockyer said that the Red Cross shelter guidance advises shelter managers to prepare for infants by having cribs and diapers available, as well as baby food, formula, and a quiet area for breastfeeding. An advocate from the U.S. Breastfeeding Committee concurred and referred participants to a physician statement on safe infant and young child feeding in disasters[5] and noted that an operational guidance document would soon be available. Breastfeeding is a resource that protects infants from gastrointestinal and respiratory diseases that are prevalent in a disaster, and lowers the infant's and mother's stress levels. In addition, it reduces the cost of managing disasters and increases community resilience. The participant also alerted shelter managers to the fact that women may want to bring their breast pumps and frozen milk supply to the shelter.

For older children, Casey-Lockyer continued, the rise in peanut allergies is a concern. The Red Cross is evaluating options such as peanut-free snack zones, placing snacks out of reach of children so they cannot help themselves, and possibly having EpiPens available in the shelters (in accordance with laws and policies). It is important to note that shelf-stable meals were designed for the dietary needs of adults in the military, and they are extremely high in sodium and calories. These meals are not suitable for a 2-year-old, Casey-Lockyer noted, or for an 82-year-old who may have the beginnings of congestive heart failure. Some companies are coming out with lower-calorie, lower-sodium meals, but sodium is a key component in the long-term preservation of the meals. Shelter managers also have the ability to purchase fresh food. Some children, especially infants, may also require tube feedings, and shelters need to be prepared.

Casey-Lockyer cautioned that although we have done well with the types of disasters we have had in the United States, we have not really had a catastrophic event in a large urban city that results in many thousands of unaccompanied minors in the suburbs. This scenario has not been addressed by school systems or shelters. How will we sustain children for extended periods, and how are we going to reunite parents who were in the city during the event with their children in the suburbs?

---

[5]Available at http://www.usbreastfeeding.org/Portals/0/Position-Statements/Emergencies-Statement-2011-USBC.pdf (accessed September 9, 2013).

Providing Child Care in Shelters

After a disaster, children suffer from a kind of benign neglect, said Judy Bezon, former associate director of Children's Disaster Services (CDS), which is part of Church of the Brethren Disaster Ministries. Children are confused and do not understand what is going on around them, Bezon said. They may see their parents crying, worry about who will take care of them, where their pet is, and why they cannot go home. They have very little control over their environment, have few coping skills, and are completely dependent on others for recovery. Young children also have limited language, and limited conceptual skills. They do not think to ask questions to get the reassurance that they might need from parents, and parents are often so totally consumed with their own worries that they do not have the emotional ability to reach out to their children and find out what is going on with them. Bezon reiterated that the mistaken perception is that if they are playing, they must be doing fine.

Children have concerns, she said, and these are often expressed and worked out through play. Adults may see children playing, and play is normal, so they assume the children are carefree and not impacted by the disaster. As an example, she described how a young girl in a FEMA facility after Hurricane Katrina had been playing with a doll and when she left the staff noticed that she had carefully raised the doll bed up on toy blocks, presumable to protect the doll from the flooding that she had experienced. She also described a brother and sister at a facility in Joplin who used empty boxes to build a "tornado-proof house." Children's drawing can also be quite telling. Following the tornadoes in Oklahoma, center volunteers reported using up the dark colors of tempera paint as the children were painting tornadoes and storms.

Children's Disaster Services

Because children use play to express themselves and to understand their experiences, CDS volunteers use a comfort kit full of toys that promote imaginative play. This is a very safe medium, Bezon explained. Children process the disaster experience at their own pace and in a safe environment using their own language and the natural language of play. If the children are too worried or not ready to deal with the disaster on their own or through the play, they will play about stereotypical things. CDS has about 600 volunteers nationwide, and they are trained to follow the child's lead in play. Volunteers participate in a 27-hour experiential workshop, staying overnight in a simulated staff shelter to give them a sense of what families are going through, as well as what they will go through if they need to stay in a staff shelter during a disaster. The training emphasizes the social and emotional phases of a disaster, rather than the impact, response, recovery, and long-term recovery. They learn to interact with children after a disaster and how to communicate through play, and they undergo a very rigorous screening process to be certified to work with children.

CDS's work in shelters and service centers allows parents to attend to business, such as applying for aid and other recovery activities, without having their children with them. This is an important resource for parents because life is disrupted for many families and their former child care arrangements, including babysitters and family members, may no longer be options. Parents can also leave children with the volunteers at CDS simply to get a break from the "hyper vigilance" needed in a crowded shelter environment to take a much needed shower or nap. Volunteers are also trained to talk with the parents about their concerns regarding their children.

Partner agencies (e.g., FEMA, Red Cross, local groups) report that CDS creates an environment that makes it easier to give aid to those in need, Bezon said. "By offering child center care, emotional support and a sense of normalcy, the CDS program helps to meet the immediate needs of children, assists family members who may be overwhelmed as they attempt to deal with the effects of the disaster, and plays an important role in fostering resiliency among children" (Peek et al., 2008, p. 408).

BEST PRACTICES AND POTENTIAL STRATEGIES DURING RESPONSE

Moving from high-level conversation from involved organizations on different operational needs, this section shifts focus to tactics and practices already being used on the ground in different sectors. Because children make up such a large percentage of vulnerable populations, it is important to continue to integrate their needs across planning areas and situational scenarios. Speakers describe examples of patient tracking, accessible evacuation planning, and hospital-level pediatric competency exercises in the next section.

Best Practice Examples from the Texas Department of State Services

Bruce Clements, director of the community preparedness section of the Texas Department of State Services, said that Texas has the largest number of federally declared disasters of any state in the nation. Events the Department has responded to since 2007 include hurricanes, wildfires, disease outbreaks (West Nile virus, tuberculosis, measles, mumps, H1N1 influenza), foodborne illness outbreaks, the plant explosion in West, Texas, and the raid on the Yearning for Zion Ranch. The Department also activated in response to a spike in hospitalizations of young women with mercury poisoning, which turned out to be from mercury-tainted skin cream from across the border. A growing issue for Texas is the need to shelter unaccompanied minors. The thousands of unaccompanied children who cross the border from Mexico are returned home according to a reciprocity agreement with the Mexican government, which can be as simple as filling out the forms and walking them across the bridge. However, there has been a recent surge of undocumented Central American minors who travel north to Mexico and then cross into the United States. It takes longer to arrange to return them home, and they need to be sheltered in the interim. Clements noted that Texas contracts with BCFS for most of its shelters across the state.

Texas is continually threatened by hurricanes and tropical storms, and Clements pointed out that the capacity the state has built to respond to hurricanes is very flexible and scalable, and has enabled the response to other events. Texas has had "a lot of practice with a lot of diverse types of threats," Clements said, and he shared several of the state's best practices and initiatives in four key areas: regional preparedness, infection prevention, sheltering, and tracking.

Local and Regional Pediatric Preparedness Initiative

Clements highlighted the Houston Regional Healthcare Pediatric Preparedness initiative as one of the best in the state, in part because of the lessons learned from a long history of flooding and from the city's role as a central location for evacuees from Hurricane Katrina.

Houston's pediatric disaster planning includes, for example, a prophylaxis dispensing form that has weight conversion charts; pre-identified pediatric response teams to assist at National Disaster Medical

System reception sites; pediatrics patient inclusion in exercises; and preparedness guides for families from the children's hospitals in the area.

Another resource from the Houston initiative is the "Together Against the Weather" website with videos and information on how to prepare for a hurricane, whether evacuating or sheltering in place. There is information for people with access and functional needs (e.g., the elderly, individuals with disabilities, developmentally disabled children), and public service materials for emergency management personnel, social services, and the media.

Houston has also expanded pediatric preparedness training to all the health care providers in the area, and provides quick reference materials, such as the Broselow Pediatric Emergency Tape, for pediatric medications, doses, equipment, etc.

Infection Prevention

The concurrent threats posed by the first cases of H1N1 pandemic influenza in late April 2009, and the start of hurricane season that June, raised serious concerns about infection prevention during evacuation and sheltering. In preparation, two different infection control kits were developed, one for buses and one for shelters (see Box 7-2). Although designed to address the double threat of H1N1 and hurricane season, Clements said these kits are now in regular use.

BOX 7-2
Contents of Infection Control Kits

Bus Kit

- Surgical masks
- Hand sanitizer
- Trash bags
- Nonlatex gloves
- Disinfectant wipes
- Disinfectant spray
- Alcohol wipes
- Tissues

Shelter Kit

- N95 respirators
- Surgical masks
- Exam gowns
- Nonlatex gloves
- Disinfectant wipes
- Disinfectant spray
- Alcohol wipes
- Tissues

SOURCE: Clements presentation, June 11, 2013.

Pediatric Sheltering

Sheltering planning for children in Texas is focused in the full range of pediatric vulnerability, Clements said, medical, behavioral health, and social (also referred to as biopsychosocial). The biggest challenge is variability across the state with the integration of the three elements. The quality of the preparedness plans that are already in place is also a concern. Although there are requirements for schools, child care facilities, and foster families to have disaster plans, there is no quality check on those plans, or criteria to define quality, Clements said. This is an important gap to be addressed, and an opportunity for very-high-risk populations to get fundamental support.

Clements pointed out that state laws and definitions differ regarding the "age of childhood" (NLCHP, 2012). The majority of jurisdictions define childhood as under the age of 18; however, for several it is under 17 or 16 years of age. Some laws also bifurcate youth and children (e.g., someone up to the age of 12 is a child, and someone aged 13 to 18 is a youth), and in some jurisdictions childhood or youth may encompass persons older than 18. These laws impact both general population and medical sheltering. In most cases a person needs to be 18 years or older to consent to medical care, but in Rhode Island, South Carolina, or Texas the age is 16; in Alabama, Hawaii, and Indiana it is 14; and in Guam and Puerto Rico anyone below the age of 18 can consent if he or she is married. If a child is separated from his or her family, short of surgery, the child can generally make decisions on whether care is received.

Multidisciplinary teams are involved in pediatric sheltering planning in Texas. Among those included are child life specialists who assist with coping, normalization, and play therapy; and Child Protective Services, especially those who are conservatorship specialists and can assist with emergency orders for medical consent. Clements added that all members of the multidisciplinary team need to have at least basic incident command training. Texas also promotes crisis counseling skills for responders, and uses the psychological first aid field guide from the National Child Traumatic Stress Network.[6]

---

[6] The *Psychological First Aid Field Operations Guide* is available at http://www.nctsu.org/content/psychological-first-aid (accessed September 9, 2103).

Pediatric Tracking

There were more than 1,000 children missing in Louisiana after Hurricane Katrina, Clements said. This motivated responders from Texas who were involved in the response to Katrina to champion a banding tracking program for Texas. Using computers, a Web-based program, and barcode scanners, evacuees are given a yellow wristband with a barcode on it and a radio-frequency identification (RFID) chip inside. Personal information is entered into the system, which can be as simple as swiping a driver's license if available. Pets and medical assets are also tagged with the same RFID chip so they can be associated with the person. Portals with RFID chip readers, or staff with handheld readers, can be set up at shelter entrances, the front of a bus, or anywhere else. Evacuees can then be tracked as they board and exit a bus, or enter and leave a triage site, shelter, or medical facility. In addition to tracking individuals, manifests can be printed listing all of the people on a particular bus or in a particular facility at any given time. Clements added that they work to build trust with the undocumented population along the U.S.-Mexico border so that they are not hesitant to participate in the program. Trust is fostered through medical outreach such as an annual exercise where clinics are set up in the Rio Grande Valley offering free health care to these individuals. The banding system is a simple program that can be used across different platforms to share information during a disaster, and Clements said it has been a very successful system for Texas.

During the discussion, a participant said that after Hurricane Sandy, he was made aware that some people who were in the shelters were feeling stigmatized because when they were out of the shelter during the day they were known as being shelter residents by their wristbands. Clements responded that he had not encountered significant pushback from shelter residents thus far, and he felt that the benefits of the wristband tracking outweigh the potential for stigma. Tatro added that in Texas, no one is required to be banded, and that education and outreach have helped foster acceptance.

Evacuation and Transportation of Children with Disabilities

Richard Devylder, senior advisor for accessible transportation at the U.S. Department of Transportation, shared his perspective on best practices for addressing the needs of children with disabilities in evacuation planning. Identifying needs is the first essential step, he said, and administrators and parents often have different views on what those needs are. Next, it is important to define what resources are available, and what resources need to be brought in to help a specific child. Other key considerations in planning are the accessibility of vehicles and facilities, and ensuring access to any adaptive equipment the child may use (e.g., moving it with the child, moving it separately and tracking it, providing it onsite). If a child has a custom wheelchair designed for his or her needs, for example, simply providing another wheelchair is not suitable, and could be detrimental.

Many children with disabilities will have an individual education plan (IEP) with their school, and Devylder stressed that the child's evacuation plan should be part of his or her IEP. He also emphasized the importance of including the child in the planning process when old enough to provide input. It is the child who knows what works and does not work for him or her during drills or other events at school. There also may be certain adults that children do not trust to help them, he added, and planners need to respect that.

Evacuation plans need to include student medical information, including diagnosis, medication allergies, hazardous conditions (e.g., impact of smoke on the child and mitigating measures to take), cardiopulmonary resuscitation and defibrillator steps to take, and climate control needs. Other necessary information includes contact information for parents and guardians, doctors, and hospitals familiar with the child, so that first responders know which hospitals are best to take the child to. Devylder recommended that someone from the local fire department and law enforcement participate in the planning so that they are aware of the child's situation and how to assist him or her through the evacuation process.

Information on communication with the student during the emergency is also an essential component of the plan. Not just primary language, but how to communicate with a child with autism, a deaf child, or how to guide someone who is blind or has impaired vision. Devylder explained that someone who is blind or has low vision cannot simply be put into a wheelchair or evacuation chair as this can be extremely frightening for them. Adhering to the normal ways of communicating with that child on campus is best. An evacuation plan should also include primary, secondary, and tertiary options for exiting the building, determined by accessibility and class location. The plan should also describe under what circumstances elevators and/or evacuation chairs can be utilized. He noted that evacuation chairs vary; some can go both up and down stairs, others can only descend stairs. He also stressed that a plan must include what to do with the child after using an evacuation chair as they are extremely uncomfortable and the child cannot be left in the chair for more than 10 or 15 minutes, or risk injury. Once evacuated, how is the student transported off campus in both medical and non-medical emergency situations? The plan can include transport memoranda of understanding that define the potential use of school transportation and public transport, as well as private entities (e.g., community partners, shuttles, taxis).

Children with disabilities need support teams, including an evacuation team, a primary education team, and a substitute team, each with at least three people assigned, Devylder said. If the child had an aide assigned, the aide should also have a defined role in evacuation. The evacuation team should include someone who is very familiar with the child, usually a school nurse, counselor, or teacher who will be available to be with the child and to make decisions during the evacuation of the child (i.e., the lead should not be a teacher who is also responsible for other children in a classroom). With the plan in place, training and drills are essential. "To know it is to do it," Devylder concluded.

Competency in Pediatric Disaster Training and Education

Jeff Upperman, program director for the Pediatric Disaster Resource Training Center (PDRTC) at the Children's Hospital Los Angeles, described novel teaching techniques implemented with the support of Hospital Preparedness Program (HPP) funding. Los Angeles is about 4,000 square miles, with a population of about 11 million, including 2.5 million children below the age of 18. Children's Hospital Los Angeles has about 300 beds, and there are approximately 400 pediatric beds total in the County of Los Angeles. The PDRTC is part of a disaster network that includes multiple hospitals; however, as the only hospital dedicated to pediatric needs in Los Angeles County, the center is the county resource on pediatric disaster preparedness. It is the hub supporting many spokes, Upperman said.

Upperman defined competence, or competency, as the ability of an individual to do a job properly, whether it is care, leadership, or management. But in developing competencies, we often train people for a certain period of time, give them a paper test, and send them off. When conducting drills and exercises, especially hospital-based, are we really seeing if care providers can intubate in austere conditions? Can they recognize posttraumatic stress disorder and other mental health issues? It is important to train and practice, but there also needs to be some level of competency, he said.

A leader in the community helps to make the community resilient and is a role model. Leaders at work (i.e., on commissions, committees, etc.) agitate the system, providing leadership for those who cannot provide it for themselves, such as children. Managers implement the plans through drills and exercises. What competencies are necessary to make these things happen?

Upperman highlighted several tools that PDRTC developed with the support of HPP to help foster competency in disaster response. The first is a prototype disaster preparedness logistics tool for pediatric emergency decision support (Neches et al., 2009). The software was designed for hospitals in Los Angeles County to use to begin thinking about their specific plans based on their specific needs. They could, for example, enter a zip code in Los Angeles County into the system and learn, based on available census data, how many children live in that zone and what might be the expected impact to the neighborhood during an earthquake.

A novel approach to education is games which allow people to practice what they have learned. Working with the University of Southern California Games Institute, PDRTC developed an online game, Surge World, to give health care workers practice in triage, resource management, and preparedness planning.[7] Another example described by Upperman was the "Disaster Olympix," an interactive drill to foster communication, collaboration, and leadership (Goodhue et al., 2010).[8] Fire teams, engineers, pediatricians, nurses, and others at Children's Hospital Los Angeles participated in competitive events testing their knowledge, skills, and abilities to respond to disaster situations. Finally, Upperman described a tri-hospital drill using technology, including robots and telemedicine, to facilitate triage and treatment consultation by offsite pediatric specialists (Burke et al., 2012).[9] In closing, Upperman

[7]Surge World is available to play online at http://lachildrenshospital.net/SurgeWorld (accessed September 9, 2013).

[8]Upperman played a brief video of the Disaster Olympix, which is available at http://www.youtube.com/watch?v=sZVgdRj-bCc (accessed September 9, 2013).

[9]Upperman played a brief video showing the use of telemedicine robots during the drill which is available at http://www.youtube.com/watch?v=sqfZI7Vqsh8 (accessed September 9, 2013).

urged participants to lead, innovate, and evaluate. Thinking about the specific needs of children and families in shelter situations prior to an emergency, and utilizing and encouraging best practices from other cities, can continually improve both the mass care operations and surge capacity at area hospitals that may not typically care for children.

8

Monitoring Children's Mental Health After Disasters

Highlights of Points Made by Individual Speakers

- Anyone who interacts with children after a disaster can be a potential source of assistance and support. However, if they are unprepared or insensitive, they can be a source of further distress.
- A single disaster event is really part of a cascade of other events in a child's life and results in cumulative impact and stress, even if the prior events are completely unrelated.
- Stigma related to mental health is a still barrier, even in times of national crisis.
- Between 30 and 40 percent of a direct survivor population are at risk for developing a new disorder that they did not have until the index event.
- Traumatic grief is different from the experience of grief in other situations and requires different treatment.

Supporting the mental and behavioral health needs of children in disasters was a recurring statement throughout the workshop. The speakers in this section of the report focused on heightened triage and targeting of vulnerable children for intervention more than demonstrating effective interventions. However, it should be noted that there are not enough data in this area to prove interventions are successful after traumatic events. Definitive guidance requires far more research on the comparative effectiveness of interventions targeting children exposed to traumatic events (Forman-Hoffman et al., 2013). Although earlier chapters covered some of the behavioral health implications for local planners, this section goes deeper into mental health needs and manifestations in children during their recovery period. In addition to a focus on coping and post-disaster processing, there is also the presentation of a tool that schools and other organizations can use to monitor and triage mental health needs in their population.

ENSURING THAT CHILDREN ARE COPING

David Schonfeld, director of the National Center for School Crisis and Bereavement, shared his list of key points for short-term mental health response for children. First, pediatric health care providers play a critical role in the mental health response to disaster. On a daily basis, pediatricians and other pediatric primary care providers are the de facto mental health providers for children in this country. Children are most likely to receive treatment from their primary care physicians for mental health disorders and psychosocial problems, which Schonfeld noted are actually the most common chronic conditions seen in pediatric practices. In the aftermath of a disaster, primary care providers are likely to be the first, and possibly the only responders to provide mental health services to children.

Adults who work with children should understand the likely reactions to disaster and know techniques to help them cope, Schonfeld continued. This includes psychoeducation and supportive services to accelerate the natural healing process. Different types of staff have different relationships with children and can offer different perspectives. As an example, Schonfeld noted that it was cafeteria workers who noticed that girls had been cutting themselves in reaction to a school shooting in which a classmate was killed. They could see this because the girls' long sleeves would pull back as they reached out with their lunch trays to be served, revealing the cuts on their arms. Anyone who interacts with children after a disaster can be a potential source of assistance and support but, unfortunately, he said, if they are unprepared or insensitive, they can be a source of further distress.

Helping children necessarily includes helping their families and communities as well. For example, parents may need help to take care of themselves in order to be able to be more available to take care of their children. Helping children also means helping health care providers to fulfill their roles. Professional staff members have their own basic needs, and crisis preparedness and response plans need to consider the professional's needs as a priority. These professionals may be impacted directly themselves and may have some of the same behavioral and mental health needs as those they serve. Professional self-care is important, but is often neglected. It is distressing to be with children who are in distress. It is critical that staff find ways to have their own personal needs met, and appreciate and address the impact of supporting children who are grieving or traumatized.

Understanding the Timeline of Recovery

Beyond the immediate response, we need to appreciate the timeline for recovery, Schonfeld said. Everyone has a baseline level of function with some highs and lows (see Figure 8-1). When a disaster event occurs people feel vulnerable, their usual coping mechanisms may fail, and they may feel helplessness and hopelessness. As communities respond and provide resources, people start to have improved functioning. This is still a vulnerable period, Schonfeld stressed. Some individuals continue their recovery and return to their baseline functioning, and some even have "posttraumatic growth" and achieve a new baseline of even higher level functioning. But others never return to their original baseline and live in a state of continued impairment. There is often an increase in suicides in this period. Unfortunately, Schonfeld said, children are thought of as "resilient" and support is often withdrawn as soon as there are signs of recovery. Instead, they need to be supported until they return to their baseline level of functioning.

The scope of need is broad, and there is a wide range of reactions and concerns beyond the acute trauma and posttraumatic stress from a disaster. For some children, bereavement is a primary issue if they have lost someone close to them. Other children face a cascade of secondary losses and stressors such as loss of their homes and relocation, loss of their peer network, difficulty integrating into new social networks or bullying at their new school, academic failure, financial stresses on the family, and parental stress, depression, substance use, or increased domestic violence. Schonfeld also pointed out that a single disaster event is really part of a cascade of other events in a child's life and results in cumulative impact and stress, even if the prior events are completely unrelated. When responding to one event, we are responding to all of the events in the life of the child. As an example, Schonfeld said that after a busload of children went through a decontamination process for minor exposure to a noxious substance, most children retuned to baseline functioning rapidly, but two girls continued to display significant stress. Further investigation revealed that one had recently seen a family member murdered and the other was being abused at home. Schonfeld also suggested that health care providers need to alter their practice patterns to include trauma history in the overall patient history.

Psychosocial Needs and Stigma

Another point Schonfeld raised is that stigma related to mental health is a still barrier, even in times of national crisis. Parents may not seek assistance because they often underestimate symptoms in their children, or they assume the children are just having normal reactions to abnormal events and professionals would not be interested. Children may withhold complaints because of concerns that they are abnormal, or they want to protect their parents who are visibly upset.

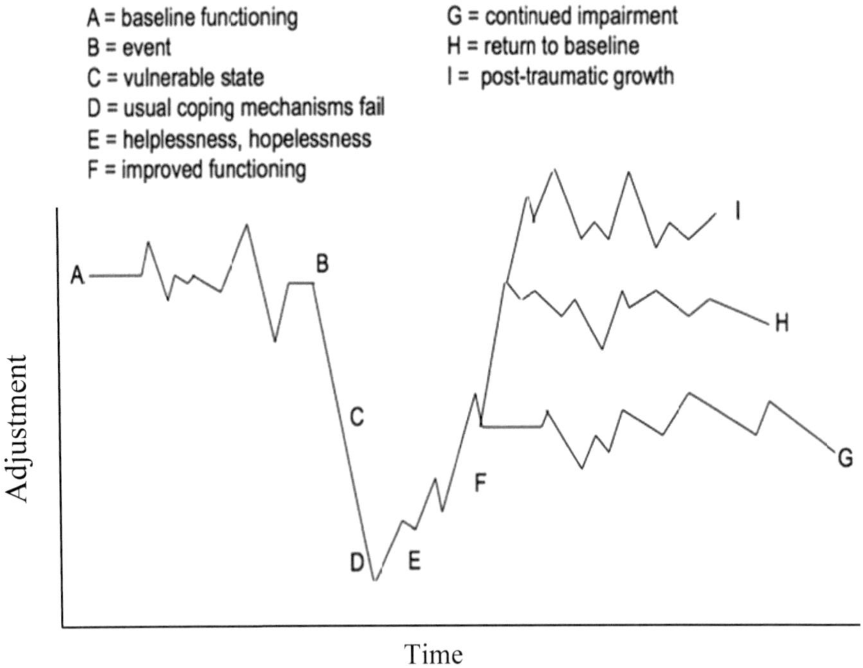

FIGURE 8-1 Adjustment over time in a crisis situation.
SOURCE: Schonfeld presentation, June 11, 2013.

Schonfeld reemphasized the work of the National Centers for Disaster Medicine and Public Health which is developing online training materials that can be used more broadly by the general public, including a module on attending to the psychosocial needs of children. He also mentioned a project with the American Federation of Teachers, the National Education Association, the National Association for School Psychologists, and others, to create materials that would be disseminated to all of their memberships. There are many materials being developed, but facilitating the dissemination and uptake of those materials is a challenge, and he recommended working through professional organizations. Roth urged that the training materials being developed also be made accessible for those with varying needs (e.g., captions on video materials, e-book device accessible).

TRIAGING HIGH-RISK CHILDREN

Merritt Schreiber, director of psychological programs at the Center for Disaster Medicine of the University of California, Irvine, School of Medicine, described a national children's disaster mental health concept of operations (NCDMH CONOPS) that he developed with funding from the Terrorism and Disaster Center of the National Child Traumatic Stress Network (Schreiber, 2011).

A very large subset of people, including children, experience transitory distress (e.g., insomnia, fears of recurrence, fears of separation). For many, resilience happens without any intervention. However, between 30 and 40 percent of a direct survivor population are at risk for developing a new disorder that they did not have until the index event (posttraumatic stress disorder [PTSD] being the most common). The concept of operations is designed to get to that high-risk subject in a timely way, and offer them evidence-based interventions that have been shown, through randomized controlled studies, to have an impact. The goal is a seamless continuum of triage-to-care incident operation. Schreiber said that there is a critical window at 30 to 45 days post-event in which intervention can reduce or even prevent clinical PTSD. Timely intervention may also reduce the secondary mental health burden on both emergency departments and primary care settings.

Included in the NCDMH CONOPS is the PsySTART Rapid Mental Health Triage and Incident Management System. PsySTART does not measure symptoms (as symptom measurement in acute aftermath of an event is often unreliable) and is not a diagnostic measure. Rather, it measures exposure, traumatic loss, early emergence of potentially ongoing or persistent stressors, disaster-related injury and illness, and peri-traumatic panic. A triage form prompts staff to collect information from individuals about their experiences (e.g., psychological panic symptom, direct life threat, exposure, trapped, saw bodies, had direct loss of loved ones, home loss). The responses help identify which patients need to be seen first.

Aggregated individual PsySTART data can be used to estimate site-level and population-level impacts of a disaster and develop a total picture of risk (types, locations, number of children at risk). Geographic information system mapping of data from multiple sites enables a common operating picture and near-real-time situational awareness of children's mental health needs. This is then used to guide incident management, define needs, allocate resources, and facilitate interagency coordination. Schreiber noted that a PsySTART mobile app has recently been developed.

In closing, Schreiber referred participants to another resource from the National Child Traumatic Stress Network, a trauma-focused cognitive behavioral therapy online training course.[1] He described it as a high-end intervention for the very-high-risk subset who are not likely to progress to resilience without intervention. Traumatic grief is different from the experience of grief in other situations, he said, and requires different treatment. Triaging high-risk children, while also taking into account important trauma histories and exposure to other incidents can be instrumental in ensuring that children progress through a recovery of timeline along with their peers, and return to their normal baseline after an event or reach further growth potential.

[1]Available at http://tfcbt.musc.edu (accessed September 9, 2013).

9

Fostering Recovery Through Community Resilience

Highlights of Points Made by Individual Speakers

- To be resilient, people, systems, and the infrastructure that supports those systems have to work together simultaneously to return to normal, whether that is the original state of normal, or a new normal.
- A capabilities-based approach to disaster preparedness develops core disaster response capabilities that can be deployed across a wide range of situations (rather than creating new plans, equipment, and responses for every disaster).
- Factors impacting resilience or the associated trauma in children include dose (magnitude of the situation), context, developmental period when exposure occurs, association with a capable caregiver, self-efficacy, and resilience of families and other systems.
- A child's resilience is embedded not just in the child, but also in the relationships, culture, and all the other communities and systems the child may interact with.
- Schools are part of the community continuum, and teachers and child care workers are first responders. They should be trained on the typical responses and needs of children by age and development.
- Older children and youth can be provided with manageable but meaningful roles in recovery.
- The unfortunate onset of a disaster creates a critical moment to leverage the media on children's behalf, show the challenges that communities face, and advocate for policy changes.

Presidential Policy Directive 8 (PPD-8) on national preparedness "is aimed at strengthening the security and resilience of the United States through systematic preparation for the threats that pose the greatest risk to the security of the Nation."[1] As defined in PPD-8, resilience is "the ability to adapt to changing conditions and withstand and rapidly recover from disruption due to emergencies." Session chair Kathryn Brinsfield, formerly of the White House National Security Staff and now the Acting Assistant Secretary for Health Affairs at the Department of Homeland Security, said that to really be resilient, people, systems, and the infrastructure that supports those systems, have to work together simultaneously to return to normal, whether that is the original state of things, or a new normal. PPD-8 takes a capabilities-based approach to disaster preparedness. The intent is not have new plans, equipment, and responses for every disaster, but to have core disaster response capabilities that can be deployed across a wide range of situations.

To further consider resilience interventions in children from a scientific perspective, a white paper was commissioned for the workshop and presented in this section. David Abramson, deputy director of the National Center for Disaster Preparedness at Columbia University, presented an overview of the white paper "The Science and Practice of Resilience Interventions for Children Exposed to Disasters."[2] The paper, authored by Abramson, Kallin Brooks, and Lori Peek, provides a review of the current literature on resilience research, and identifies several challenges to developing an evidence base for resilience interventions in disasters. Following first a discussion of research on the science of resilience in children, and then an explanation of the white paper, panelists provide real-world examples of specific strategies to foster resilience.

THE FOUNDATIONS OF RESEARCH ON RESILIENCE IN CHILDREN AND YOUTH

Ann S. Masten, of the Institute of Child Development at the University of Minnesota, said that the field of disaster research and awareness was motivated in large part by the incredible global devastation from World War II, and the millions of traumatized children impacted by bombings, radiation, displacement, and being orphaned.

---

[1] See http://www.dhs.gov/presidential-policy-directive-8-national-preparedness (accessed September 9, 2013).

[2] Full text of the white paper is available in Appendix G of this workshop summary and online at http://iom.edu/~/media/Files/Activity%20Files/PublicHealth/MedPrep/2013-JUN-10/White%20paper%20Abramson%20child%20resilience.pdf (accessed September 9, 2103). The authors are solely responsible for the content of the white paper.

Researchers in psychiatry, psychology, and other fields wanted to understand the impact of these kinds of experiences on child development, and what could be done to prevent problems and promote better development in children with these experiences.

Factors That Impact the Resilience of Children

Masten highlighted several of the top factors that impact the resilience of children in a disaster. Dose is key, not just the magnitude of the current situation but also prior exposure to adversity, ongoing adversities that often cascade following a mass trauma experience, and cumulative adversity. There is also much interest now in toxic stressors that can alter health, well-being, or epigenetic status in the long term. This also reinforces David Schonfeld's earlier point clarifying that response to one event in a child's life is actually a response to all of the events in that child's life, and having providers maintain trauma histories can be helpful in understanding a child's response to a singular event and how it might be impacted from previous stressors.

Other experiences of great adversity in children's lives are relevant to understanding disaster, but context matters a great deal. Context matters not just in terms of the history and the nature of the exposures, but also the recovery context. One of the most powerful predictors of how children will do is to track the quality of the recovery context, she said.

Masten cited a growing recognition of sensitive periods in the course of development when children are more susceptible to certain kinds of exposures (e.g., radiation, toxins associated with disaster, traumatic stress). These exposures can be experienced directly by the child, or prenatally because the pregnant mother is experiencing severe trauma and stress. Studies in Finland in the aftermath of Chernobyl, for example, are showing biological sequelae in children who were prenatally exposed not to the radiation, but to the extreme fear and stress experienced by the mother during pregnancy. Many aspects of a child's risk exposure, resources, and response capabilities are dependent on where the child is developmentally. Expectations of children and how they are going to be able to handle stress also varies developmentally as well as culturally. Individual differences, ranging from genetic variations to personality differences, impact how a child might interact with disaster experiences.

Neurobiology now has the tools to study epigenetic change and intergenerational transmission of trauma effects.

A large literature on resources and protective factors suggests that one of the most important factors for children to help them deal with adversity is a capable care giver. Self-efficacy is also important because it is attached to the motivational system that drives people to try to cope in the midst of adverse situations. Children also depend on the resilience of families and of many other systems.

Resilience as a Dynamic Systems Concept

The capacity for resilience is distributed across multiple, adaptive, interacting systems, Masten stressed. A child's resilience is not just embedded in the child, but also in the relationships, culture, and all the other communities and systems the child may interact with (Sapienza and Masten, 2011). The capacity for resilience in a disaster is interdependent with resilience in other kinds of systems (e.g., economic resilience, global resilience in terms of climate change).

Masten emphasized that many systems influence the capacity that children have for resilience. Systems in the organism (i.e., the child) include, for example, the immune system, stress response systems, central nervous system, cognitive skills, executive functions, and motivation. Much of child capacity is also embedded in relationships. Secure attachment relationships with young children are with caregivers, but as we get older, attachment expands to friends, mentors, romantic partners, and to spiritual relationships (e.g., with a pastor or religious leader). Other systems in communities and societies that are important for children include schools as well as the emergency response systems, health care systems, and cultural practices.

To foster resilience in children, general guidelines from the literature are to plan developmentally, target and time interventions strategically, consider multiple levels of action, define and prepare first responders, and promote resilience of key systems for children. With regard to planning, Masten said to prepare for children medically, psychologically, and pragmatically. Recognize that teachers and child care workers are first responders, and train them on the typical responses and needs of children by age and development. Masten also noted that many first responders are parents, and they are likely to perform better if their own children are safe and protected.

The resilience literature also argues for reducing and mitigating risk. One way to promote better outcomes is to reduce or avoid exposure to risk, she said. For example, avoid separation of children from their attachment figures; monitor exposure of children to adversities, including the media; reduce stress of pregnant mothers; and help parents to regulate negative emotion. Other strategies emphasize the importance of restoring routine systems that symbolize normalcy to children, such as family meals, school and play opportunities, and cultural and religious practices. Support the natural and familiar helpers (families, school, and teachers) and adaptive systems in a child's normal environment so they can support and comfort children. Masten also reiterated the points made by Houston and others about providing older children and youth with meaningful but manageable roles in recovery.

Resilience is common, and does not require anything special, Masten concluded. There is more than one way to achieve resilience, and given a favorable recovery context, most children will recover. The needs, vulnerabilities, and strengths of children vary individually, and by development, situation, and culture. Recovery depends on very fundamental adaptive systems (within the child, in relationships, and in the systems), and restoring and protecting these systems are high priorities.

THE SCIENCE AND PRACTICE OF RESILIENCE INTERVENTIONS FOR CHILDREN EXPOSED TO DISASTERS

Abramson cited the work of Wright and colleagues who classified the existing research on resilience into "four waves": identifying individual factors associated with resilience; understanding how those factors develop as processes in complex systems; understanding how to foster resilience (i.e., interventions); and understanding the biology and the epigenetics of resilience (Wright et al., 2013). In conducting their research, the authors sought to address four key questions: What is the long-term impact of disasters on children and youth, and how does it relate to resilience and recovery? What does a resilience trajectory look like? How does one balance promoting positive traits and protecting against pathophysiological states? How can resilience be activated?

What Is the Long-Term Impact of Disasters on Children and Youth and How Does It Relate to Resilience and Recovery?

Abramson highlighted three overarching findings regarding exposure to disasters, impacts, and recovery. First, disasters may be only a moment in time, but they exert a long-term enduring effect on children and youth. "Toxic stressors" may extend the effects of a disaster into the adult years, leading to complex comorbidities. Abramson referred participants to the Institute of Medicine and National Research Council report *From Neurons to Neighborhoods* for more information about the impact of toxic stressors on children (IOM and NRC, 2000). In addition to the stress of the disaster, the child may have other acute or chronic stresses in their life, as mentioned previously, and the effects can be cumulative. Second, children are embedded in larger social systems and their health and well-being is highly contingent on functioning support systems in their lives (e.g., parents, households, schools, community institutions, neighborhoods). And third, children and youth often want to be actively engaged in their own recovery.

Gulf Coast Child and Family Health Study

As an illustration, Abramson described the Gulf Coast Child and Family Health Study conducted from 2006 through 2010. This longitudinal cohort study followed 1,079 randomly sampled households in Louisiana and Mississippi for up to 5 years after Hurricane Katrina (including 427 households with children). During the course of the study, the percent of children living in a trailer or a hotel declined from 83.8 percent in 2006 to 7.5 percent in 2010. However, the percent of parents who reported that they were not coping well was consistently between 13 and 20 percent. Parents with mental health distress declined from 61 percent to 43 percent; however, Abramson noted that more than 40 percent of parents exhibiting mental health distress after 5 years is still an enormous number. Parents who felt their children were not safe in school remained high, at 25 to 37 percent. And more than half reported moving in the past year in the 2010 survey.

Abramson next considered what systems in the children's lives had an effect on their mental health. Children were directly impacted by parental constraints such as mental health distress, inadequate social supports, minimal sense of community, or lack of a sense of "life recovery." Household stressors accounted for the most effect (e.g., unstable housing, loss of income, not enough money for food, poor family functioning). Social stressors in the neighborhoods also had a statistically significant and substantial effect on the child's mental health (e.g., drug sales, prostitution, gangs and crime, signs of vacancy). Interestingly, prior social adversity had no statistical effect. Almost 5 years after Hurricane Katrina, Katrina-affected children and youth had rates of serious emotional disturbance that was five times the national average of a comparable group. Understanding these long-term impacts can help inform resilience interventions, and recovery expectations, Abramson said.

What Does a Resilience Trajectory Look Like?

Developing a resilience trajectory (i.e., plotting the ability to withstand, adapt to, or recover from a disaster event) is hampered by the limited availability of pre- and post-disaster data, and the lack of defined and standardized resilience outcomes measures. Outcomes could be, for example, the percentage of children without pathophysiology, the percentage at an age-appropriate grade, or the percentage with a subjective sense of "stability." However, there are issues with all of these outcome measures. For example, many children are too old for their grade in school because the family has been displaced and they did not attend school or attended sporadically, or the family is in a new school system that is more rigorous than the school system they came from, and they are behind. Subjective measures are impacted by bias, Abramson noted, and parents often underreport their children's problems.

How Does One Balance Promoting Positive Traits and Protecting Against Pathophysiological States?

Resilience-based efforts are designed to promote optimal development in children, Abramson explained. Approaches used seek to enhance their healthy and adaptive cognitive, emotional, and social processes, and to develop their skills in solving problems, expressing emotions, and forming relationships. These promotional efforts often take place before a disaster, so that they can be activated after the child has been exposed to the stressor. Symptom-based efforts are employed to

BOX 9-1
Key Protective and Promotive Factors Highlighted by David Abramson

- Positive self-identity (self-efficacy; self-worth and self-esteem)
- Executive control and self-regulation
- Coping skills (problem-solving competence; stress reduction)
- Supportive relationships (parents, siblings, peers, trusted adults)
- Opportunities for "pro-social behavior" (helping others)
- Positive worldview (hopefulness; faith; communal solidarity; contextualized understanding of hazard/catastrophe)
- Stability (parental, household, institutional, communal, social routines)

reduce or address mental health problems. Approaches focus on decreasing psychological symptoms through individual and group therapies; using graded exposure and inoculation strategies to decrease stress; and applying "meaning making" to the stressors to help contextualize what the children have experienced (Peltonen and Palosaari, 2013).

Resilience- and symptom-based efforts can complement each other. By enhancing resilience-based efforts, we may be able to avoid stress-induced mental health symptoms. By addressing mental health problems resulting from stress, Abramson said, we may be able to achieve optimal development and resilience (see Box 9-1).

How Can Resilience Be Activated in Children?

Abramson summarized four ways that children's resilience can be "activated." Many times, it is through extemporaneous policy decisions. For example, the Joplin School District made the decision to open 87 days after the tornado that devastated 6 of their 10 school buildings. This was an immediate and clear policy decision that was not governed by other preexisting policy decisions or plans, and it set a very clear objective for recovery (discussed further by Besendorfer below).

Another approach is through policy advocacy and community engagement. Save the Children's Program on Resilient and Ready Communities, for example, works to ensure that the emergency operations plans in a community have taken into account all of the child institutions, promoting policy infrastructure so that decisions do not have to be made extemporaneously (discussed further by Spangler below). The Communities Advancing Resilience Toolkit is similar, but takes more of an asset building approach, Abramson explained.

A third way to activate resilience in children is through programs and interventions. Abramson divided these into two basic categories: pre-disaster moderators as primary prevention for those who may be exposed (e.g., preparedness education, stress reduction training, public health) and risk-activated moderators as secondary prevention for those who were exposed (e.g., Vietnamese American Young Leaders Association [VAYLA] and Rethinkers, discussed further below).

Finally, resilience can be activated through providers and the workforce. The Joplin Child Care Taskforce, for example, is working to train providers in the community to address many of the psychological needs the children are facing.

He offered several examples of programs that increase self-efficacy, including the Masters of Disaster curriculum of the American Red Cross, Boy Scouts and Girl Scouts preparedness badges and awards, the Wisconsin Responding to Emergencies and Disasters with Youth (READY) camp and classes, Teen Citizen Emergency Response Team (CERT), and the Youth Council at the Federal Emergency Management Agency (FEMA) (the latter discussed by Houston in Chapter 6). These are very similar, Abramson said, in that they all occur before the disaster, and focus on building skills and self-efficacy.

Promoting Positive Worldview in Children

The white paper research also identified several examples of projects that promote a positive worldview after a disaster. The New York City–based 9/12 Generation Project is a day of volunteer service held on 9/12 (i.e., the day after 9/11). VAYLA was established in New Orleans after Hurricane Katrina to fight a toxic waste dump that was going to be located in their neighborhood, and has since evolved into a robust youth engagement and empowerment initiative in New Orleans for youth of all race and ethnicities. The Urban Resilience Program in Israel is very targeted toward preparation for terrorism in an effort to provide stress reduction.

Abramson elaborated on the Rethinkers program, which promotes both a positive worldview and empowerment. Rethinkers was started as a summer program in the aftermath of Hurricane Katrina, with 20 middle school students in New Orleans. The students were charged with helping to find solutions to fix the problems in their schools. The students surveyed more than 500 other children from a sampling of schools in New Orleans on issues that matter to students. The Rethinkers have produced reports, held press conferences, and made recommendations to the city, some of which have been acted on. They have also led campaigns to make changes to bathrooms, cafeterias and food, and discipline policies. They have now expanded to rethink nutrition, weight and obesity issues, architecture, digital media, food justice, gardens, and restorative justice.

Challenges to Building an Evidence Base on Resilience in Children

The authors of the white paper identified three major types of challenges to the development of an evidence base for resilience interventions: definitional, operational, and political. The definition of resilience is a topic of considerable debate, as can be understood by the varying definitions from different sources in this report alone. Is it a process, an outcome, or a latent construct? Is it the presence of a positive state, or the absence of a pathological state? Most scholars would agree, Abramson said, that resilience only manifests in the face of a stressor. How can you determine baseline resilience of a community if resilience can only be measured in the presence of the stressor. Operationally, disasters are rare and unpredictable events and the factors underlying resilience are complex, multilevel systems (biological, psychosocial, social, cultural). Finally, from a political perspective, the federal government, which is the largest purchaser of academic research, does not generally fund direct resilience intervention services, so it has little reason to fund resilience research. Most of the resilience program funding comes from the nonprofit and philanthropic sectors, which have little surplus for funding research, Abramson said. In addition, many of the issues around resilience are “root cause” problems, social problems such as health disparities and social inequities, for which there is limited political advocacy especially in the face of constrained budgets.

From Research to Action

In closing, Abramson described the Gulf Coast Population Impact Project as a case example of how research moves to action.[3] The project objective was to characterize the ways that the Deepwater Horizon oil spill affected children in communities along the Gulf Coast, and to identify resources and services that would most benefit these children.

Secondary data were used to develop an oil spill impact score and identify heavily impacted communities. Researchers then interviewed 1,437 parents in Alabama, Florida, Louisiana, and Mississippi regarding exposure to the oil spill, and physical or mental health effects. Focus groups were also conducted with children, caregivers, health care providers, educators, and community leaders.

The data showed that poverty and exposure to the oil spill were most statistically significant factors in well-being. Key health and wellness themes that emerged from community engagement were lack of access to care (especially for mental health), clusters of unexplained symptoms (e.g., nose bleeds, ear bleeds, skin rashes), unsupervised children and unsafe behavior, and dwindling recreational and occupational opportunities. Participants in the focus groups also cited economic pressures and cascading stressors (e.g., not enough food, parental depression, eroding cultures) and the inability of the community to sustain economic opportunities, social programs, and provider networks. For many communities, Hurricane Katrina and the oil spill were not really two disasters, but one long continuous disaster, with acute stressors layering on top of chronic stressors. Abramson relayed that in one of the fishing communities, 1 out of every 11 girls in the high school was pregnant. According to a local community leader, "the only thing to do around is go fishing, get high, or get pregnant, and we can't go fishing anymore."

This data compelled the researchers to take action and the SHOREline (Skills, Hope, Opportunity, Recovery, and Engagement) youth empowerment project was developed. The goal is to build a network of high school chapters that will develop and enhance their agency, self-efficacy, positive worldview, and pro-social behavior. Youth help other youth recover from disasters. The project does not ask the youth about themselves, Abramson explained, but rather, how can they help others in their families and communities. This resilience

---

[3]Children's Health after the Oil Spill: A Four-State Study Findings from the Gulf Coast Population Impact (GCPI) Project—http://academiccommons.columbia.edu/item/ac:156715 (accessed November 12, 2013).

intervention will be measured, and reported on in the future, Abramson concluded.

PROMISING PRACTICES OF CHILD-SERVING PARTNERS

After discussing resilience research highlights and concepts from Masten's research and identified in Abramson's white paper, the summary now shifts to on the ground case studies of resilience examples in children and best practices in disasters. Because this area is still new and evolving, it is somewhat of a moving target, but continual sharing of strategies and communication across sectors—again broadening stakeholders—can help develop understanding of children in this vulnerable state.

Joplin Schools as an Example of Resiliency

Angie Besendorfer, assistant superintendent for the Joplin (Missouri) Public School District, began her presentation with a safety message urging everyone to reevaluate their school tornado shelter plans, in particular, to find safe areas other than interior hallways (where students have traditionally been taught to line up and duck and cover). Security cameras that were still functioning when the tornado hit the Joplin school buildings on Sunday, May 22, 2011, show that those hallways became wind tunnels where equipment and soda machines went flying.[4] Had the tornado been on a school day, she said, "it would have been horrific."

Besendorfer played a brief news video to show some of what the city of Joplin experienced. Three thousand of the approximately 7,700 students lived in the direct path of the storm. Seven students and 1 school staff member were killed, and 4,200 students were without a school at the end of the storm. Nine schools and the administration building were hit by the tornado, six of which were a total loss. Around the city, 8,000 homes, 400 business, and 18,000 vehicles were damaged or destroyed, and 161 community members were killed.

Prior to the storm, the school district was already on a first-name basis with city leaders, chamber leaders, and federal and state

[4]The security camera footage can be viewed on the school district website at http://www.jet14ondemand.com/ondemand/musicvideo.php?vid=9974a0414 (accessed September 9, 2013).

representatives. Also in place was the Bright Futures Initiative, a network which links business, social services agencies, and faith-based partners to schools. The district also had strong communications strategies, including social media, phone calling systems, a website, and relationships with media outlets. According to Besendorfer, having these aspects already in place greatly benefited the school system's resiliency and recovery.

The immediate response focused on finding people from the total school family of about 9,000 employees and students. Outreach was done through social media, teachers' relationships with students and parents, phone calls, media, and simply walking the neighborhoods. The district felt that it was important to provide some sort of closure, and with 12 days left in the school calendar, the school year was declared finished and an event was held at every school, whether it was standing or not. These were set up as celebrations to start the summer, Besendorfer said, but they offered closure and let children, families, and teachers see each other and know that they were all okay. Another aspect of the immediate response was attending the funerals of the students who passed, and the family members of students, being there to support the children in their tragic losses.

Importance of Establishing and Meeting Expectations

Besendorfer explained that the school district established a clear goal immediately following the storm; school would start again on August 17 of that year, just 84 days after the tornado hit. In addition, summer school was started on time and for the first time, it was extended through July and transportation was provided (as many parents had lost their cars). Summer session was really one way to provide a safe place to be for students who needed it, and although the program was for elementary students, middle school and high school students could serve as helpers.

Temporary education facilities were set up in leased spaces, for example, in the mall. Progress on the creation of spaces was shared through the media. It was important to reassure the community that there were going to be quality places for their children to attend school, so that people would stay in Joplin and recover together. The district stressed the message that it might be a temporary location, but it was not a temporary education. Groups of students toured the facilities so that they could share the progress with their friends and foster excitement about starting school. This was particularly important for the high school students who lost their school and wanted to quit. But when they came to see the facility at the mall, unlike anything they had had before, and learned they were going to get laptops, there was renewed interest. The short-term response also included taking care of the adults. All administration and staff at the hardest-hit schools were required to have a 30-minute visit with the counselor.

Additional support was provided during the course of the 2011-2012 school year. In partnership with the Ozark Center from Freeman Hospital, counselors and caseworkers were embedded in all of the schools in the district, not just those damaged by the tornado, because everyone was ultimately impacted. Besendorfer noted that they were originally called trauma counselors, but they were renamed "hope counselors." Another intervention was Winter Camp during Christmas break, again, for students who needed somewhere safe to go. The district also worked with the governor and FEMA to create a playground and a community building in the FEMA village. Mercy Hospital hosted community dinners twice per month at the schools to help bring people from the neighborhoods back together. Finally, the "Sunshine Squad" was a group of people who would come to a school and do something for the kids, and then something for the teachers, just to "lighten the air."

Looking Forward

For the school year 2012-2013, the hope counselors are continuing in the schools through a grant. Besendorfer noted that there were even more counseling needs in the second year after the tornado, and there was currently no funding for year three, although several grant applications had been submitted. Also in the second year, all of the school counselors received Cognitive Behavior Therapy in Schools (CBTS) training. Three thousand students are still in temporary schools while replacement schools are under construction. Besendorfer added that all of the temporary school sites and the schools that were affected have temporary storm shelters, and safe room additions are being added to all of the elementary schools (with mitigation funding through Sections 404 and 406 of the Stafford Act).

In summarizing her overview of Joplin schools as an example of resiliency, Besendorfer said that schools are part of the community continuum, and having a relationship with the whole community is very important. Approaches that were successful included setting clear goals and making them very public. This creates accountability but also gives people hope. Celebrating frequently is also critically important. Celebrating the opening of school, the first football game, or ground-breaking for new schools helped children to make the positive presupposition that everything was going to be all right, and helped them to behave as if it was. The schools became a part of the community pride. Perhaps the most important asset to recovery, she concluded, has been the school staff, and she closed with a video of staff and students telling their stories of resiliency and hope.[5]

Save the Children

Save the Children was founded in England in 1919, established in the United States in 1933, and now works in more than 120 countries around the globe. Kathy Spangler, vice president of U.S. programs for Save the Children, said that in the United States, it is the leading advocate and responder for children in emergencies. Save the Children is working to mobilize communities in all 50 states to better protect children in emergencies through federal and state advocacy, and policy change. Toward this end, the organization produces an annual national report card that provides a state-by-state assessment of school and child care emergency planning for evacuation, reunification, meeting functional and mobility needs, and multiple disasters. States are ranked on their policies each year, and Spangler said that currently, only 17 states meet the very minimal requirements in all four areas. Spangler reiterated the theme expressed by others that the unfortunate onset of a disaster creates a critical moment to leverage the media to speak on children's behalf, to show the challenges that communities face in meeting their needs, and to advocate for much needed policy changes.

Children's Task Forces

One of the best practices shared by Spangler is the establishment of a Children's Task Force. First used by Save the Children in 2005 in New Orleans in the aftermath of Hurricane Katrina, the convening of a children's task force is now institutionalized in the immediate response to a disaster. The task force engages key stakeholders, including federal, state, and local partners and nongovernmental organizations, to prioritize

---

[5]The video can be seen at http://www.youtube.com/watch?v=XF-rWJKdgCE (accessed September 9, 2013).

the response and recovery needs of children and child-serving programs. A related best practice is the establishment of a working group (a subset of the task force) to focus on child care recovery. The sooner child care can be operational again, the sooner families can get back to work and get reestablished in their communities. A key challenge to making a rapid assessment of the impact of a disaster on child care is the lack of any central database or registry of facilities, Spangler said.

For Hurricane Sandy, three task forces were established, for New Jersey and New York at the state level, and for New York City. Save the Children is planning to continue its work with Hurricane Sandy recovery through June 2014. Following the immediate response, the organization's focus has shifted to child care recovery. Save the Children has awarded around 200 recovery grants to child care facilities in New York and New Jersey. Save the Children is also partnering to provide its Journey of Hope psychosocial recovery program to children and their caregivers. Because the tornadoes in Moore, Oklahoma, were in May, at the end of the school year, the focus there was also on child care recovery, as well as expansion of summer camp programs. Grants to local organizations such as the YMCA facilitated free attendance at camp for more than 350 children in affected communities.

Emergency Planning and Response Programs

Another best practice highlighted by Spangler is the Child-Friendly Spaces program, which is the organization's key emergency response program. It meets immediate needs by setting up care and activities for children in shelters and other places where families congregate during disasters. By the end of 2012, Child-Friendly Spaces had served 1,485 children in 16 Hurricane Sandy shelters. Child-Friendly Spaces were also set up within 6 hours of the Sandy Hook Elementary shooting in Newtown, Connecticut, and operated for more than 2 weeks in conjunction with crisis counseling services for families.

Save the Children has also developed the Resilient and Ready Communities Initiative, a national program to improve community planning to protect children in emergencies. Resilient and Ready Communities was born out of Save the Children's work across six high-risk regions in the United States. It is focused on systems building, and core elements of the initiative have been utilized at the state and local levels, and in large urban and small rural settings. Trainings to build local capacity to protect children in emergencies have been provided in communities of all sizes in all 50 states through webinars and online learning. Spangler noted that Resilient and Ready has been recognized by the J. Getty Trust and the American Red Cross as a strategy that has brought together disparate systems into a more organized capacity-building approach.

The six key components of the initiative are (1) engaging key stakeholders through training, awareness raising, and advocacy; (2) assessing current capacity and monitoring progress; (3) informing practice and emergency planning improvements; (4) evaluating resiliency post-disaster; (5) renewing and refreshing resiliency through continuous improvement; and (6) mobilizing communities in support of children's protection through relationship building and meaningful engagement. As examples of activities in these core areas, Spangler said that Save the Children is currently working with Columbia University to develop a child-focused preparedness assessment tool to help communities identify gaps and focus areas. The organization is also working in a number of county-level jurisdictions in California to draft children's annexes to their emergency management plans.

Although it's clear that defining and understanding resilience in children is difficult, especially in the wake of a disaster during their developmental years, continued research and case studies from youth groups and child advocacy organizations from around the country can help to identify best practices and tactics children need to recover from adverse events. Engaging youth groups and looking at cross-sector outreach between public health professionals in health equity, social justice, and disaster risk reduction could show new ways of achieving a similar goal of building a stronger community where children can grow.

10

Hurricane Sandy Experience: Disaster Recovery Focused on Children and Families

Highlights of Points Made by Individual Speakers

- The federal government's role in recovery is to support locally led recovery efforts to restore and improve the health care and social services networks in the affected communities.
- The health and the human services functions of the Department of Health and Human Services (HHS) need to work in tandem, educating each other about their respective disciples, and communicating better about available tools and resources.
- The goal of a children's task force is to develop a common operating picture on children's needs across the public, education, and early childhood sectors.
- A key aspect of the response to Hurricane Sandy was coalition building though the activation of existing resources and relationships.
- A barrier to response and recovery efforts for child care is that there are thousands of independent operators who are not part of organized networks, and are not reachable through standard communication mechanisms.
- An all-hazards approach to planning and training for child care providers includes chain of command, communications, emergency kits, evacuation and sheltering plans, and business recovery.

In the final chapter on recovery, panelists discussed examples of human services disaster recovery interventions that promote the social and economic well-being of children and families in the aftermath of disasters. The "recovery" phase begins almost as soon as the disaster and response end, but it continues for long after the rest of the country stops watching. Monitoring children and families during this recovery phase is critical and has often been overlooked. With the release of the Federal

Emergency Management Agency's (FEMA's) National Disaster Recovery Framework (NDRF), there is more focus and guidance for this important phase of rebuilding communities, and monitoring of social and economic determinants can give great insight to the process. During both the response and recovery phases, it is important to highlight the need for coordinated communication and action from the many players involved related to children. With a lack of power and communication options immediately after the storm, as well as jurisdictions responding differently based on their state or city protocols, streamlined activity and information gathering across child care providers can remain a difficult challenge. Representatives from state and federal level children and family agencies highlight their experiences during and after Hurricane Sandy hit the East Coast in October 2012.

NATIONAL DISASTER RECOVERY FRAMEWORK: HEALTH AND SOCIAL SERVICES RECOVERY SUPPORT FUNCTION

Joyce Thomas, regional administrator for Administration for Children and Families (ACF) Region II,[1] described the NDRF as the federal structure for how to best restore, redevelop, and revitalize the health, social, economic, natural, and environmental fabric of the community following a disaster. The NDRF defines the roles and responsibilities of the federal government in recovery, and provides guidance on coordinating structure, recovery planning, and building stronger, smarter, and safer communities.[2]

The NDRF established six recovery support functions (RSFs) that provide a structure to facilitate the identification, coordination, and delivery of federal assistance to supplement the state, local, private, and nonprofit efforts in affected communities. The RSFs are community planning and capacity building; economic; health and social services; housing; infrastructure systems; and natural and cultural resources. Each RSF has coordinating and primary federal agencies, and supporting organizations.

The coordinating agency for the health and social services RSF is the Department of Health and Human Services (HHS), with the Office of the

---

[1]Region II includes New Jersey, New York, Puerto Rico, and the U.S. Virgin Islands.

[2]The National Disaster Recovery Framework is available from FEMA at http://www.fema.gov/national-disaster-recovery-framework (accessed September 9, 2103).

Assistant Secretary for Preparedness and Response (ASPR) as the lead. The federal government role is to support locally led recovery efforts to restore and improve the health care and social services networks in the affected communities. Core mission areas include health care services impacts, social services impacts, referral to social services/ disaster case management, public health, behavioral health impacts, environmental health impacts, food safety and regulated medical products, animal health, school impacts, and long-term health issues specific to responders.

ACF's Role in Emergencies

ACF, through the Office of Human Services Emergency Preparedness and Response (OHSEPR) and in collaboration with each of 10 regional offices, provides national leadership in human services preparedness, response, and recovery. ACF is focused on child well-being, and Thomas said that ACF services touch the lives of every community and every tribal nation across the country.

In the event of any major disaster, ACF

- provides situational awareness on human services systems status and disaster-caused unmet needs;
- conducts outreach to Office of Child Care (OCC) and Office of Head Start (OHS) programs and grantees;
- coordinates federal support for children's needs;
- conducts immediate disaster case management assessments and services;
- participates in the identification of the "problem set" for federal partners;
- defines the landscape of potential need for federal support and engagement across interagency in support of health and social services recovery, including new partners coming in to assist in response and recovery;
- focuses on establishing structure to support local long-term recovery operations at regional level; and
- identifies opportunities for building resilience (capacity, mitigation).

As an example of ACF activities, Thomas highlighted the role of ACF in support of the health and social service RSF core mission area of referral to social services/disaster case management. ACF implements coordinated systems for rapid referral to appropriate social services, and strategic leveraging of federal service programs to mitigate social disruption and transition people back to self-sufficiency. ACF also facilitates the Federal Disaster Case Management program to address unmet recovery needs.

Hurricane Sandy and the NDRF

Hurricane Sandy was the first large-scale event that prompted NDRF implementation, Thomas said. The storm impacted 5 of the 10 ACF regional offices. About 70 staff members were deployed during the response phase, logging more than 16,000 staff hours. Three disaster case management assessments were conducted, which indicated that 86 Head Start centers and 697 child care centers were closed across Connecticut, New Jersey, and New York.

In the transition from response to the recovery phase, ACF provides recovery-related technical assistance for HHS and ACF programs by encouraging, facilitating, and supporting children's task forces; providing support from OCC and OHS for early childhood center re-openings; providing early childhood programs and children's issues subject matter expert teams; and providing linkages to human services networks. In addition, ACF provides financial recovery assistance through Social Services Block Grants, Head Start funding, and Family Violence Prevention Grants. Thomas noted that ACF provided $474 million in funding for Hurricane Sandy recovery, $2 million of which will go toward family violence prevention. An additional $95 million in recovery aid will be available for Head Start centers.

In closing, Thomas stressed that the health and human services pieces of HHS need to work in tandem, educating each other about their respective disciples, and communicating better about available tools and resources. Unlike a disaster event, recovery is a process and may take a very long time. Restoration of health and social services systems following a disaster requires coordination, communication, and collaboration among various levels of government, nongovernmental organizations (NGOs), and impacted communities. Situations such as Hurricane Sandy provide teachable moments, and Thomas reiterated the need to seize those moments to make change and make the lessons learned become future actions. She urged participants not to become weary in doing good and important work.

CHILDREN, YOUTH, AND FAMILIES TASK FORCES FOR RECOVERY

Lieutenant Commander Jonathan White, deputy director of the Office of Human Services Emergency Preparedness and Response at ACF within HHS, stressed that responding to the needs of children in disasters is not about "pediatric populations" or "at-risk populations." It is about children, youth, and families, and the world as children encounter it. It is vital, he said, to have a strategy that is multisectoral and multidisciplinary.

White highlighted three key challenges to meeting the needs of children, youth, and families in a disaster. One of the foremost challenges is the limited interoperability of human services, public health and medical (including behavioral health), and emergency management systems. Of these three areas, White noted that human services is least connected to the other two. Second is the profound vulnerabilities of child care providers and the formidable financial barriers to child care recovery. White explained that a public hospital that suffers an uninsured loss looks to FEMA for public assistance. However, as for-profit entities, the vast majority of America's child care providers are ineligible for FEMA public assistance. Many are also ineligible for Small Business Administration disaster loans because their profit margins are too small to make them credit-worthy. As noted earlier, child care workers are not well funded at baseline, with average earnings of about $21,000 per year. Third, disaster human services in the United States have historically focused on sheltered populations, not communities; however, the human services purview is the entire population.

> "As for-profit entities, the vast majority of America's child care providers are ineligible for FEMA public assistance. Many are also ineligible for Small Business Administration disaster loans because their profit margins are too small to make them credit-worthy."
> —Jonathan White

Community-Level Task Forces

A key intervention, White said, is the community-level task force focused on children, youth, and families' needs in recovery. The task force is a whole-community coordination forum that is multisectoral, multilevel, and multidisciplinary. It is often led by a state agency with equities in children's services, convened by the state with support from ACF and Save the Children, and brings together a broad array of child-serving organizations (see Box 10-1).

The goal of the task force is to develop a common operating picture on children's needs across the public, education, and early childhood sectors. A key feature of the task force is that it makes available to community-level leaders a ready channel to get technical assistance and subject-matter expertise from national organizations and federal agencies. The task force facilitates the integration of early childhood programs and the behavioral health mission. One of the most important places to be providing behavioral health services in the birth-to-5 age group is child care and Head Start, he said. The task force also enables resource pooling to address gaps. In Joplin, Missouri, for example, the tornado struck just after the Head Start centers in that community had closed in the summer. Head Start grantees had transportation and facilities that were child-suitable and were able to add these resources to the pool and help close the care gaps in the remainder of the community.

Because of the particular vulnerabilities of child care, White said it is often helpful to have a child care workgroup within the larger children's task force. Participants would include the lead state agency for child care (in some states there may be multiple lead state agencies for child care), ACF, the child care resource and referral agency, Save the Children, child care providers, affected families, FEMA, and others.

The role for national organizations and federal agencies in recovery is to support the state leadership, empower communities, and provide them every resource and tool that will help them achieve recovery. The community needs ownership of the process, White concluded.

BOX 10-1
Examples of Individuals and Organizations That Participate as Task Force Members

- State agencies with children's services equities
- Affected parents and youth
- Child care providers
- Child care resource and referral agencies
- Child welfare agencies
- Behavioral health agencies
- Individual pediatricians, pediatric nurses, social workers, child psychologists, child life specialists
- After-school care providers
- Recreational services programs
- Runaway and homeless youth providers
- Family violence prevention and services agencies
- Agencies serving children with disabilities
- Public health and environmental health authorities
- Schools (principals, teachers, counselors, social workers)
- Local religious leaders
- Community action agencies
- Head Start providers
- National Voluntary Organizations Active in Disasters (VOAD) focused on children (e.g., Save the Children, Southern Baptists, Church of the Brethren Children's Disaster Services)
- Child advocate organizations
- Federal partners including ACF, ASPR, FEMA, others as needed (e.g., Small Business Association, HUD, EPA)

NOTE: ACF = Administration for Children and Families, ASPR = Office of the Assistant Secretary for Preparedness and Response, EPA = Environmental Protection Agency, FEMA = Federal Emergency Management Agency, HUD = Department of Housing and Urban Development.
SOURCE: White presentation, June 11, 2013.

STATE PERSPECTIVE: NEW JERSEY CHILD TASK FORCE

Allison Blake, commissioner of the New Jersey Department of Children and Families (DCF), discussed preparedness and response before, during, and after Hurricane Sandy. In the state of New Jersey, DCF is responsible for Child Protective Services, all of children's behavioral health care, and services for children with intellectual and developmental disabilities. DCF operates a network of special education schools for pregnant and parenting teens and children with profound physical impairments, and a very large network of community-based family-strengthening child abuse prevention programs. Blake noted that DCF has no responsibility or authority for sheltering or decision making around mass care. Each of the 21 counties in New Jersey has a county department of human services that is responsible for emergency sheltering and for local homeless sheltering and boarding homes; a county department of health; and an office of emergency management. In each county, there is also a board of social services (formerly called the county welfare agency) that provides temporary assistance for needy families, emergency assistance, and housing assistance. In some counties, the head of Social Services reports to the Department of Human Services, while in others it operates independently. This inconsistency across counties became one of the most complicated parts of the disaster response to Hurricane Sandy, Blake noted.

Preparations

Hurricane Sandy touched down in New Jersey on October 29, 2012. Blake said that the magnitude of the approaching storm was not fully appreciated until 4 or 5 days before that. In preparation, DCF looked to other jurisdictions for lessons about child welfare. For example, when Hurricane Katrina hit Louisiana in 2005, many state offices were impacted. At that time, Louisiana did not have a client tracking system or a robust system of electronic records, and numerous paper records were destroyed or lost. As a result, foster children who moved out of state with their displaced foster parents were essentially missing, for 2 years in some cases. Medications and prescriptions were lost for children in foster care (and many of the children in the welfare system are taking psychotropic medications which should not be discontinued abruptly).

In fall 2012, New Jersey already had a robust electronic record system in place for case management. In preparation for the storm, DCF established the existing child abuse hotline as the hub or central point of communications for contact with DCF on any issue. All children's and women's service providers and all foster parents were notified of this central contact hub via blast e-mails, phone calls, and alerts on the DCF website. Staff were sent to coastal areas to retrieve state vehicles used to transport children and move them to higher ground so they would be serviceable after the storm.

After the Storm

Devastating flooding and widespread power outages meant that many people did not have television or Internet access to obtain news. The DCF central operations, where the hotline is based, did not flood or lose power, and it became the central point of communications and operations. DCF was able to put in calls to every foster parent in the state within the first 5 days after the storm. There were also daily conference calls with FEMA and the Red Cross.

The day after the storm, the governor's office began holding conference calls twice daily and providing reports on the number of people in shelters. Although they had data on the number of adults, senior citizens, and even pets, there were no data on children in shelters. As a result, DCF sent "well-being teams" to the shelters to meet with the Red Cross and the county staff and check on the children and families. Blake explained that the name of the teams was intentionally chosen because many people hear "State Department of Children and Families" but think "Child Protective Services." Blake noted that although many individuals and families who stayed in longer-term shelters were not known to the public systems, they had been living on the edge and were in need of public services. DCF had public health nurses and social workers talking with these people to understand why they were still in the shelter after they were able to return to their communities or other housing options.

A key aspect of the response to Hurricane Sandy was coalition building though the activation of existing resources and relationships. Immediately after the storm, DCF contacted the human services directors in the impacted counties. DCF also reached out to the FEMA-operated disaster recovery centers to provide information about available local social services and community support. The State-Led Child Task Force was also created, focused on identifying a short-term recovery plan for children and families, and long-term recovery needs around trauma, resilience, and other issues. In addition to DCF and the New Jersey Departments of Health, Human Services, and Education, task force members included FEMA, ACF, AAP, New Jersey Volunteer Organizations

BOX 10-2
New Jersey DCF Long-Term Recovery Plan Target Areas of Focus

Strengthening families and preventing incidence of child abuse that would be exacerbated by the storm

- Strategically bolster DCF's network of Family Success Centers to enable the centers to continue to be a resource to families during the long-term recovery phase.
- Provide direct assistance to foster/resource homes displaced by the storm to maintain stable home environments for children under the care of the Department of Child Protection and Permanency.
- Ensure child protection worker caseload sizes remain at appropriate levels to be able to effectively and efficiently respond to allegations of abuse or neglect.
- Expand respite services for families with children with special needs.
- Engage pediatric primary health care practices in a partnership to assess, identify, and intervene in a coordinated manner to mitigate the potential negative impacts of this disaster.

Preventing violence and exploitation exacerbated by the storm's impact

- Broaden existing domestic violence prevention programming.
- Prepare the domestic violence intervention system for the expected increase in incidents of domestic violence.
- Strengthen programs for homeless youth and victims of human trafficking.

Building resiliency and supporting recovery

- Expand access to mental health services for children.
- Provide evidence-based psychosocial disaster recovery programming in schools.
- Provide psychosocial programming for child care centers and other early childhood centers to promote positive early childhood development and build resilience.

SOURCE: Blake presentation, June 10, 2013.

Active in Disaster (VOAD), Montclair State University, Save the Children, and others. Blake stressed the importance of recognizing the unique needs of the local jurisdictions. DCF worked with the county long-term recovery committees to understand the greatest need and gaps in their communities. In January 2013, DCF issued a report on the state's long-term recovery plan, which is focused on keeping families strong, preventing the potential negative impacts of the disaster on children and families, and providing swift support and intervention (see Box 10-2).[3] Next steps for the state include gathering additional stakeholder feedback, tracking and adjusting in coordination with coalitions, and preparing for the upcoming hurricane season with the new working group and coalition in place.

NEW YORK STATE CHILD CARE RESPONSE

The New York State Office of Children and Family Services (OCFS) is the child welfare agency, the juvenile justice agency, and regulates all modalities of child care (with the exception of child care centers in New York City). Janice Molnar, deputy commissioner of the Division of Child Care Services at the New York State OCFS, described the office's preparation and response to Hurricane Sandy.

There are more than 4 million children in New York State, and almost 400,000 live in the Hurricane Sandy surge areas.[4] In the days before the storm, OCFS staff prepared geographic information system (GIS) maps of all of the child care providers in the vulnerable coastal areas of the Rockaways and Long Beach. In the days immediately following the storm, the initial focus of OCFS was identifying child care programs that were open and possibly able to take in children from affected areas. She pointed out that this was different from the early federal data collection focus, which was on identifying programs that were closed (to make the case for resources before Congress). There are numerous challenges to collecting data from child care facilities. There are thousands of independent operators who are not part of organized networks, and often not reachable through standard communication strategies and mechanisms. Because many home-based providers are not technology-savvy or do not have e-mail, OCFS still sends out important communications by regular mail, resulting in delays in response. Staff also went door to door to conduct operational assessments of providers. The numbers of open and impacted centers was continuously refined as more information became available. Ultimately, about 11,500 licensed and registered child care programs were impacted by the storm in the 13

---

[3]Available at http://www.state.nj.us/dcf/home/HurricaneSandyRecoveryPlan.pdf (accessed September 9, 2013).

[4]See http://datacenter.aecf.org/data/tables/102-child-population-by-gender?loct=34&loct=2#detailed/2/34/false/868,867,133,38,35/14,15,65/421,422 (accessed September 9, 2013).

counties for which President Obama issued a major disaster declaration (more than half of the 21,000 regulated programs in the state as a whole).

Tools and Best Practices

The day after Hurricane Sandy, OCFS developed and implemented an assessment tool for the licensing staff to use when determining the level of impact on child care programs (via phone if possible, or on foot through onsite inspections). One of the goals of outreach, Molnar explained, was to help open programs stay open, even those without heat, running water, or light. Children's circumstances were so dire that most would not have fared any better staying at home, and for many it would have been even worse. It was also important to maintain the continuity of care for children to preserve some sense of normalcy in their lives, and to support parents who were struggling with significant issues and for whom the provision of child care was a relief. The GIS maps of facilities created before the storm were overlaid against FEMA maps of flood and surge zones so that OCFS could triage outreach to programs that had the greatest potential of being impacted on the storm. Assessors looked for very basic health and safety procedures (e.g., bottled water, safe food storage, sufficient clothing and blankets, sanitation, working smoke detectors, a way to contact emergency services, and sufficient staff/ adequate child supervision). Molnar noted that OCFS waived staff-to-child ratio and group-size requirements on a case-by-case basis to keep as many programs open as possible. She added, as noted by others, that many of the staff helping in the recovery effort were themselves impacted by the storm.

Working to Stay Open

The New York government is a state-supervised, county-administered system, which means that the 62 counties have a considerable authority in determining how they run their child care subsidy systems and other social services. Because there was no time for counties to do plan amendments, OCFS created a simple checklist that counties could submit (by e-mail or by phone) for on-the-spot approval by the state of expanded services to affected families. Districts could be allowed, for example, to extend the eligibility period for services, expand the definition of a child needing protective services, or expand the amount of time a district can pay for child care for families seeking employment. Molnar stressed the importance of daily communication with the commissioners of the departments of Social Services in the affected counties, representatives of the governor's office, and representatives of all applicable state agencies.

In addition to outreach, OCFS co-chairs the Children's Issues Task Force with ACF Region II (discussed by Thomas, above), and Molnar noted that they continue to meet monthly. Meeting agendas included topics such as review of time sensitive deadlines, update on temporary shelters and assistance, updates on housing, or mental health supports. Subcommittees concentrate on specific topical areas such as outreach to immigrant populations, disaster-related food loss, and behavioral and mental health.

OCFS made resources for providers and families available on its website in both English and Spanish, issued waivers to programs to allow them to temporarily relocate, and OCFS staff provided onsite case management at the seven FEMA disaster recovery centers on Long Island. In addition, Governor Cuomo issued an executive order that allowed for temporary suspension of certain statutory provisions related to programs under the jurisdiction of OCFS (for example, child care subsidy eligibility predetermination could be processed in the absence of a family's supporting documents, which were likely destroyed in the storm).

Lessons Learned

Molnar described current OCFS activities to improve child care provider emergency preparedness. Existing regulations are very basic and require providers to have a written plan for evacuation and to have evacuation drills once per month. OCFS is proposing new regulations to ensure that each program has onsite supplies sufficient for an overnight stay, including nonperishable food, water, first aid, and other safety equipment in the event parents are unable to pick up children due to a local disaster. There is also a focus on all-hazards planning and training for providers, including chain of command, communications, emergency kits, evacuation and sheltering plans, and business recovery. Online videos are available for providers on emergency scenarios such as what to pack in a "to go" bag or emergency kit.[5] It can take a while for actual on-the-ground practice to catch up with best practice, Molnar concluded, and in New York "we've had no choice but to catch up as best we can."

As national guidelines and support at the federal level are beginning to include the "recovery" phase more and more in documents and agendas, these children and family agencies affected by Hurricane Sandy are important examples of the work and outreach that need to be done after the incident occurs. This also presents an opportunity to engage child care providers and agencies across the country to share lessons and work collectively through ACF on improving plans and preparedness for future incidents.

[5]The video library is available at http://www.ecetp.albany.edu/videolibrary.shtm#emergencyvids (accessed September 9, 2013).

11

Final Remarks

Workshop committee chair Michael Anderson noted that we are past the starting line and have made progress in many areas related to children's needs, but still need to get to a better state. The participation of national leaders and subject-matter experts was a key strength of this Institute of Medicine workshop, as was the broad array of topics discussed relevant to taking better care of children faced with disaster, he continued. Despite the diversity of experts in the room, Anderson again reiterated that there is still the need to bring others to the table and broaden the group of stakeholders that engages in these conversations at the national and local levels (e.g., more involvement from the child care and education fields, private practitioners). Many nontraditional partners familiar with children could bring a wealth of knowledge to the public health and health care professionals to augment planning and response, but they are often not engaged, or do not realize they could be a resource.

Many of the barriers to progress that were discussed are financial as well as a lack of centralization and coordination for information and resources. As noted by many participants, there is usually no payment or reimbursement for preparedness activities. Administrators and child services providers are increasingly asked to do more with less, and although they acknowledge the importance of emergency planning, there are many competing priorities. How do advocates for children make and keep disaster preparedness for children and families a priority? The concept of multifaceted efforts (i.e., designing things to meet daily operational needs that can also meet the needs of patients during disasters) was discussed as one opportunity for progress in preparedness in the face of financial constraints. Also mentioned was balancing the wealth of resources, tools, and best practices happening at the grassroots level with the lack of coordination and centralization for these issues. Moving forward, children and family issues in preparedness could use a centralized home that practitioners and caregivers across the country can access to augment their planning.

Revisiting remarks from Irwin Redlener's keynote speech, Anderson pointed out that the challenge now is figuring out how to move from lessons learned to actions taken, actually implementing the many best practices shared by speakers. In the same vein, testing the many plans and annexes that have been developed is an important second step in making sure that they are sufficient and robust enough to perform as expected. Various speakers highlighted the need for a national exercise focused on pediatrics and surge capacity. Upperman presented promising ideas to improve competency in pediatrics and using games and drills at the hospital level to familiarize providers, but taking this to a higher level and coordinating drills across regions or across the country could be very beneficial to identifying remaining gaps in plans and seeing where strengths are.

Finally, Anderson pointed out that although the summary of the workshop will help disseminate information about the many tools, websites, and resources discussed by the participants, there remains a need for a "clearing house" for sharing information and best practices. With the continued interest and engagement of invested federal agencies mentioned throughout the summary, as well as the reauthorization of the Pandemic and All-Hazards Preparedness Act of 2013, the conditions are favorable to make strong impacts in these areas of children and families in disaster preparedness, response, and recovery.

A

References

AMA (American Medical Association). 2011. *The State-Level Economic Impact of Office-Based Physicians*. http://www.ama-assn.org/ama/pub/advocacy/state-advocacy-arc/economic-impact-study.page (accessed September 8, 2013).

ASPR (Assistant Secretary for Preparedness and Response). 2012. *Healthcare Preparedness Capabilities. National Guidance for Healthcare System Preparedness.* http://www.phe.gov/preparedness/planning/hpp/reports/documents/capabilities.pdf (accessed September 8, 2013).

Burke, R. V., B. M. Berg, P. Vee, I. Morton, A. Nager, R. Neches, R. Wetzel, and J. S. Upperman. 2012. Using robotic telecommunications to triage pediatric disaster victims. *Journal of Pediatric Surgery* 47(1):221-224.

Devereaux, A. V., J. R. Dichter, M. D. Christian, N. N. Dubler, C. E. Sandrock, J. L. Hick, T. Powell, J. A. Geiling, D. E. Amundson, T. E. Baudendistel, D. A. Braner, M. A. Klein, K. A. Berkowitz, J. R. Curtis, and L. Rubinson; Task Force for Mass Critical Care. 2008. Definitive care for the critically ill during a disaster: A framework for allocation of scarce resources in mass critical care: From a Task Force for Mass Critical Care summit meeting, January 26-27, 2007, Chicago, IL. *Chest* 133(5 Suppl):51S-66S.

Forman-Hoffman, V. L., A. J. Zolotor, J. L. McKeeman, R. Blanco, S. R. Knauer, S. W. Lloyd, J. G. Fraser, and M. Viswanathan. 2013. Comparative effectiveness of interventions for children exposed to nonrelational traumatic events. *Pediatrics* 131(3):526-539.

GAO (Government Accountability Office). 2013. *National Preparedness: Efforts to Address the Medical Needs of Children in a Chemical, Biological, Radiological, or Nuclear Incident*. GAO-13-438. http://www.gao.gov/products/GAO-13-438 (accessed September 8, 2013).

Garrett, A. L., R. Grant, P. Madrid, A. Brito, D. Abramson, and I. Redlener. 2007. Children and megadisasters: Lessons learned in the new millennium. *Advances in Pediatrics* 54:189-214.

Goodhue, C. J., R. V. Burke, S. Chambers, R. R. Ferrer, and J. S. Upperman. 2010. Disaster Olympix: A unique nursing emergency preparedness exercise. *Journal of Trauma Nursing* 17(1):5-10.

IOM. 2012. *Crisis Standards of Care: A Systems Framework for Catastrophic Disaster Response*. Washington, DC: The National Academies Press.

IOM (Institute of Medicine) and NRC (National Research Council). 2000. *From Neurons to Neighborhoods: The Science of Early Childhood Development.* Washington, DC: National Academy Press.

Kissoon, N. 2011. Deliberations and recommendations of the Pediatric Emergency Mass Critical Care Task Force: Executive summary. *Pediatric Critical Care Medicine* 12(Suppl.):S103-S108.

Lasker, R. D. 2004. *Redefining Readiness: Terrorism Planning Through the Eyes of the Public*. New York: The New York Academy of Medicine.

Masten, A. S. 2011. Resilience in children threatened by extreme adversity: Frameworks for research, practice, and translational synergy. *Development and Psychopathology* 23:141-154.

Merton, R. K. 1936. The unanticipated consequences of purposive social action. *American Sociological Review* 1(6):894-904. http://www.jstor.org/stable/2084615 (accessed September 8, 2013).

NCCD (National Commission on Children and Disasters). 2010. *Report to the President and Congress*. AHRQ Publication No. 10-M037, October 2010. Rockville, MD: Agency for Healthcare Research and Quality. http://www.ahrq.gov/prep/nccdreport (accessed September 8, 2013).

Neches, R., T. Ryutov, T. Kichkaylo, R. V. Burke, I. A. Claudius, and J. S. Upperman. 2009. Design and evaluation of a disaster preparedness logistics tool. *American Journal of Disaster Medicine* 4(6):309-320.

NLCHP (The National Law Center on Homelessness & Poverty). 2012. *Alone Without a Home: A State-By-State Review of Laws Affecting Unaccompanied Homeless Youth*. http://www.nlchp.org/content/pubs/Alone%20Without%20a%20Home,%20FINAL1.pdf (accessed September 8, 2013).

Olympia, R. P., R. Rivera, S. Heverley, U. Anyanwu, and M. Gregorits. 2010. Natural disasters and mass-casualty events affecting children and families: A description of emergency preparedness and the role of the primary care physician. *Clinical Pediatrics* 49(7):686-698.

Peek, L., J. Sutton, and J. Gump. 2008. Caring for children in the aftermath of disaster: The Church of the Brethren Children's Disaster Services Program. *Children, Youth and Environments* 18(1):408-421.

Peltonen, K., and E. Palosaari. 2013. Evidence-based resilience enhancing intervention methods for children affected by armed conflict. In *Handbook of Resilience in Children and War*, edited by C. Fernando and M. Ferrari. New York: Springer. Pp. 267-284.

Phillips, R. L., M. S. Dodoo, J. L. McCann, A. Bazemore, G. E. Fryer, L. S. Klein, M. Weitzman, and L. A. Green. 2005. *Report to the Task Force on the Care of Children by Family Physicians*. Washington, DC: Robert Graham Center.

Sapienza, J. K., and A. S. Masten. 2011. Understanding and promoting resilience in children and youth. *Current Opinion in Psychiatry* 24:267-273.

Schreiber, M. 2011. *National Children's Disaster Mental Health Concept of Operations*. Oklahoma City, OK: Terrorism and Disaster Center at the University of Oklahoma Health Sciences Center. http://community.fema.gov/gf2.ti/aw/280514/32490/PDF/-/CONOPS_FINAL_120511b.pdf (accessed September 8, 2013).

Wright, M. O., A. S. Masten, and A. J. Narayan. 2013. Resilience processes in development: Four waves of research on positive adaptation in the context of adversity. In *Handbook of Resilience in Children*, edited by S. Goldstein and R. B. Brooks. New York: Springer. Pp. 15-38.

B

Abbreviations and Acronyms

AAP	American Academy of Pediatrics
ACF	Administration for Children and Families (HHS)
ASPR	Office of the Assistant Secretary for Preparedness and Response
BARDA	Biomedical Advanced Research & Development Authority (ASPR)
CCP	Crisis Counseling Assistance and Training Program
CDC	Centers for Disease Control and Prevention
CERT	Community Emergency Response Team (FEMA)
CMS	Centers for Medicare & Medicaid Services
DDH	Disaster Distress Helpline
DHS	Department of Homeland Security
DoD	Department of Defense
DOJ	Department of Justice
EHR	electronic health record
EMS	emergency medical services
EMSC	emergency medical services for children
EPA	Environmental Protection Agency
EUA	emergency use authorization
FEMA	Federal Emergency Management Agency

GAO	Government Accountability Office
GIS	geographic information system
HHS	U.S. Department of Health and Human Services
HIPAA	Health Insurance Portability and Accountability Act of 1996
HPP	Hospital Preparedness Program
MCM	medical countermeasure
MOU	memorandum of understanding
NCCD	National Commission on Children and Disasters
NCDMPH	National Center for Disaster Medicine and Public Health
NDMS	National Disaster Medical System
NDRF	National Disaster Recovery Framework (FEMA)
NGO	nongovernmental organization
NICHD	National Institute of Child Health and Human Development
OCFS	New York State Office of Children and Family Services
OHSEPR	Office of Human Services Emergency Preparedness and Response (ACF)
PAHPA	Pandemic and All-Hazards Preparedness Act
PHEMCE	Public Health Emergency Medical Countermeasures Enterprise
PHS	Public Health Service
POD	point of distribution
PTSD	posttraumatic stress disorder
SAMHSA	Substance Abuse and Mental Health Services Administration
SNS	Strategic National Stockpile
VOAD	Volunteer Organizations Active in Disaster

C

Statement of Task

An ad hoc committee will organize a public workshop that will examine public health and medical preparedness related to children and families including children with special needs. The committee will develop the workshop agenda, select and invite speakers and discussants, and moderate the discussions. Specifically, the topics to be addressed at the workshop will include the following:

- How state and local health department emergency planning should integrate the needs of children and families.
- How child care systems should incorporate emergency planning into day-to-day operations, and how they can partner with state and local health departments.
- How public health can assist with child separation/family reunification through pre-event health education development.
- Opportunities to integrate the needs of children and families in public health readiness at the state and local level.
- What community partners would be critical for covering as many children as possible (age, ethnicity, disability status, etc.) during an emergency.
- How state and local health departments should connect with these community partners for the purposes of emergency preparedness and response.

An individually authored workshop summary will be prepared by a designated rapporteur based on the information gathered and the discussions held during the workshop.

D

Agenda

Disaster Preparedness, Response, and Recovery Considerations for Children and Families: A Workshop

June 10-11, 2013

Keck Center, Room 100
500 Fifth Street, NW
Washington DC 20001

Background:

Communities across the United States face the threat of disasters almost every day, both large and small. Children represent nearly 25 percent of the U.S. population, but current state and local preparedness plans often do not include specific considerations for pediatric populations and families. The preparedness and resilience of communities related to children will require a systems framework for disaster preparedness across traditional and nontraditional medical and public health stakeholders, including community organizations, schools, and other partners in municipal planning.

This workshop will examine medical and public health preparedness related to children and families, including children with special health care needs. The workshop will review already existing tools and frameworks that can be modified to include pediatric needs, as well as partnerships and organizations with vested interest that can be leveraged in planning to improve outcomes and allow for pediatric considerations to be integrated throughout local and state emergency plans. A special focus on resilience and recovery will highlight best practices already being employed specifically for children, and what opportunities exist to explore successful recovery strategies further.

Meeting Objectives:

- Discuss progress being made in different sectors around the country related to the 2010 National Commission Recommendations and opportunities for integrating related pediatric work into local and state planning efforts
- Discuss opportunities to augment children's benefits by leveraging existing coalitions
    - Explore coalition challenges and successes from federal, state, local, and provider perspectives
- Describe opportunities to strengthen public health partnerships to address the needs of children and families
- Understand barriers and challenges to better financial systems related to pediatric preparedness
    - Discuss importance of health care financing education among stakeholders
    - Consider strategies to reduce the financial burden on public health and health care facilities
- Emphasize different capabilities needed for mass care and sheltering to provide for families and children with special health care needs
- Examine resilience strategies that lead to successful recovery in children after a disaster
- Understand current approaches and interventions to improve recovery in children after any type of emergency or disaster

DAY ONE
June 10, 2013

8:15 a.m. Welcome and Introductions

Michael R. Anderson, *Workshop Chair*
Vice President and Chief Medical Officer, University Hospitals Case Medical Center
Chief Medical Officer, UH Rainbow Babies and Children's Hospital
Associate Professor of Pediatric Critical Care, Case Western Reserve University School of Medicine

8:30 a.m. Keynote Speaker: Highlighting the Demand for a Focus on Children and Families

Irwin Redlener
Director
National Center for Disaster Preparedness

Session I:
Progress Made/Highlights from National Commission on Children and Disasters

Session Objectives:

- Examine highlighted recommendations and gaps identified during the National Commission on Children and Disasters
- Discuss progress being made in different sectors around the country and opportunities for integrating work into local and state planning efforts

8:50 a.m. Overview of 2010 Commission Recommendations

David Schonfeld
Pediatrician-in-Chief, St. Christopher's Hospital for Children
Director, National Center for School Crisis and Bereavement

9:05 a.m. Progress of 2010 Commission Recommendations

Dan Dodgen
Director
Division for At-Risk Individuals, Behavioral Health and Community Resilience
Office of the Assistant Secretary for Preparedness and Response

9:20 a.m. Discussion with Attendees

9:35 a.m. BREAK

Session II: How Can We Leverage Health Care Coalitions for the Benefit of Children?

Session Objectives:

- Discuss opportunities to augment children's benefits by leveraging existing coalitions
- Discuss achieving duality of service delivery and level of preparedness to increase capacity every day and not just during disasters
- Explore coalition challenges and successes from federal, state, local, and provider perspectives

9:50 a.m. Session Chair: Introduction and Overview of Objectives

Andrew C. Rucks, *Planning Committee Member*
Professor, Department of Health Care Organization and Policy
School of Public Health
The University of Alabama at Birmingham

10:00 a.m. Panel Presentations: Challenges and Benefits of Regional Coalitions, How to Overcome Barriers, Best Practices

Richard Hunt
Senior Medical Advisor
National Healthcare Preparedness Programs
Office of the Assistant Secretary for Preparedness and Response

Allison Blake
Commissioner
New Jersey Department of Children and Families

Patricia Frost, *Planning Committee Member*
Director
Emergency Medical Services
Contra Costa County Health Services

George Foltin
Vice President, Clinical Services
Department of Pediatrics
Maimonides Infants & Children's Hospital

Esther Chernak
Philadelphia Area Project
Drexel School of Public Health

11:15 a.m. Discussion with Attendees

11:30 a.m. LUNCH

Session III: Opportunities for Integration of Children and Family Needs to State and Local Planning

Session Objectives:

- Discussing potential alignment of Public Health Emergency Preparedness/Hospital Preparedness Program (PHEP/HPP) capabilities with pediatric planning considerations
- Describe opportunities to strengthen public health partnerships
- Exploring cross collaboration with community agencies

12:30 p.m. Session Chair: Introduction and Overview of Objectives

Georgina Peacock, *Planning Committee Member*
Developmental-Behavioral Pediatrician
Medical Officer
Centers for Disease Control and Prevention

12:40 p.m. Panel Discussion: Benefits, Gaps and Tactics in Including Child Serving Partners in Municipal Emergency Planning

Ginny Sprang
Professor, College of Medicine Department of Psychiatry
Executive Director, UK Center on Trauma and Children

Evelyn Lyons
Emergency Medical Services for Children Manager
Division of EMS & Highway Safety Illinois Department of Public Health

Linda Smith
Deputy Assistant Secretary
Inter-Departmental Liaison for Early Childhood Development
Administration for Children and Families

1:30 p.m. Discussion with Attendees

1:45 p.m. Panel Discussion: Augmenting the Reach of Public Health Planning Through Community Action

Patricia Wright
National Director
Autism Services at Easter Seals

Peter Gudaitis
Chief Response Officer
New York Disaster Interfaith Services
Ashley Houston
Youth Preparedness Council
Citizen Corps/FEMA

2:45 p.m. Discussion with Attendees

3:05 p.m. BREAK

Session IV:
Financing Health Care for Children in Emergencies: Understanding Barriers

Session Objectives:

- Discuss importance of healthcare financing education among stakeholders
- Understand barriers and challenges to better financial systems related to pediatric preparedness
- Consider strategies to reduce the financial burden on public health and health care facilities

3:20 p.m. Session Chair: Introduction and Overview of Objectives

Importance of Education of Health Care Financing and How Its Changes Impact Organizations and Communities

John Wible (Ret.)
General Counsel
Alabama Department of Public Health

3:35 p.m. Panel Discussion: Funding and Legal Barriers Encountered and Opportunities for Enhanced Payment

Health System Policy Perspective

Gregg S. Margolis
Director
Division of Health System Policy
Department of Health and Human Services

Private Insurer Perspective

Robert W. Smith
Senior Medical Director
Central Region
UnitedHealthcare Clinical Services

Hospital Perspective

Amy Knight
Senior Vice President
Children's Hospital Association

Provider Perspective

Scott Needle, *Planning Committee Member*
Community Pediatrician
Healthcare Network of Southwest Florida

4:35 p.m. Discussion with Attendees

5:00 p.m. ADJOURN

DAY TWO
June 11, 2013

8:15 a.m. Welcome and Introduction

Michael R. Anderson, *Workshop Chair*
Vice President and Chief Medical Officer, University Hospitals Case Medical Center
Chief Medical Officer, UH Rainbow Babies and Children's Hospital
Associate Professor of Pediatric Critical Care
Case Western Reserve University School of Medicine

SESSION V:
Operationalizing Response Considerations for Children

Session Objectives:

- Discuss child and family specific needs during response phase
- Emphasize different capabilities needed for mass care and sheltering to provide for families and children with special health care needs
- Explore best practices and future strategies for comprehensive response plans related to children

8:20 a.m. Session Chair: Introduction and Overview of Objectives

Kari Tatro
Executive Vice President
Emergency Management Operations
BCFS Health and Human Services

8:35 a.m. Panel Discussion: Children and Family Needs During Mass Care/Sheltering Operations

Functional Needs Support Services

Marcie Roth
Director, Office of Disability Integration and Coordination
Federal Emergency Management Agency

Nutritional Needs and Family Reunification

Mary Casey-Lockyer
Manager, Disaster Health Services
American Red Cross

Mental Health

David Schonfeld
Pediatrician-in-Chief, St. Christopher's Hospital for Children
Director, National Center for School Crisis and Bereavement

Temporary Child Care

Judy Bezon
Former Associate Director
Children's Disaster Services

9:45 a.m. Discussion with Membership

10:10 a.m. BREAK

10:25 a.m. Panel Discussion: Existing Best Practices and Future Potential Strategies During Response

Bruce Clements, *Planning Committee Member*
Director
Community Preparedness Section
Texas Department of State Health Services

Richard Devylder
Senior Advisor for Accessible Transportation
Department of Transportation

Jeff Upperman
Program Director
Disaster Resource and Training Center
Children's Hospital Los Angeles

11:15 a.m. Discussion with Attendees

11:45 a.m. LUNCH

SESSION VI:
Fostering Recovery Through Community Resilience

Session Objectives:

- Examine resilience strategies that lead to successful recovery in children after a disaster
- Understand connections between pre-event mitigation and post-event recovery for children and families
- Discuss opportunities for employing community resilience in different community sectors

12:45 p.m. Session Chair: Introduction and Overview of Objectives

Kathryn Brinsfield
National Security Staff
The White House

1:00 p.m. White Paper Presentation: Resilient Practices and Characteristics That Lead to a Successful Recovery for Children After Disasters

David Abramson
Deputy Director
National Center for Disaster Preparedness
Assistant Professor of Clinical Sociomedical Sciences
Mailman School of Public Health

1:25 p.m. Discussion with Attendees

1:40 p.m. Panel Discussion: Promising Practices of Community Sectors Related to Children That Contribute to Successful Recoveries After Disasters

Ann S. Masten, *Planning Committee Member*
Irving B. Harris Professor of Child Development
Distinguished McKnight University Professor
Institute of Child Development
University of Minnesota, Twin Cities
Angie Besendorfer
Assistant Superintendent
Joplin Public School District
Joplin, Missouri

Kathy Spangler
Vice-President
U.S. Programs
Save the Children

2:30 p.m. Discussion with Attendees

2:50 p.m. BREAK

SESSION VII:
Disaster Recovery with a Focus on Children and Families

Session Objectives:

- Understand current approaches and interventions to improve recovery in children after any type of emergency or disaster
- Examine available data and evidenced based methods to promote children's needs
- Consider importance of measuring recovery through social and economic well-being of children

3:05 p.m. Session Chair: Introduction and Overview of Objectives

LCDR Jonathan White
Deputy Director
Office of Human Services Emergency Preparedness and Response
Administration for Children and Families

3:15 p.m. Panel Presentation: Approaches and Interventions in Disaster Recovery that Promote the Social and Economic Well-Being of Children?

Joyce Thomas
Regional Administrator
Administration for Children and Families
Region II

Janice Molnar
Deputy Commissioner
Division of Child Care Services
New York State Office of Children and Family Services

LCDR Jonathan White
Deputy Director
Office of Human Services Emergency
Preparedness and Response
Administration for Children and Families

Merritt Schreiber
Associate Clinical Professor of Emergency Medicine
Center for Disaster Medical Sciences
University of California, Irvine, School of Medicine
University of California, Irvine, Medical Center

4:15 p.m. Discussion with Attendees

4:35 p.m. Next Steps: Report from Session Chairs on Key Takeaway Messages

- What issues have not been addressed?
- How can people engage their communities to pass on lessons learned?

5:00 p.m. ADJOURN

E

Biographical Sketches of Invited Speakers and Panelists

David Abramson, Ph.D., M.P.H., is the deputy director and director of research at Columbia University's National Center for Disaster Preparedness. Dr. Abramson's areas of study include disaster recovery and resiliency, the social ecology of vulnerability, risk communication targeted at high-risk or elusive communities, and survey research on preparedness attitudes and behaviors. He is the principal investigator of the longitudinal Gulf Coast Child & Family Health Study, an examination of need and recovery among more than 1,000 randomly sampled displaced and impacted families in Louisiana and Mississippi (2006-2010), and is co-investigator of a National Institutes of Health study of the impact of the Deepwater Horizon oil spill on children's health. In addition, Dr. Abramson is leading a foundation-funded effort to identify pediatric needs along the Gulf Coast. Other current or recent disaster-related research activities include studies of how U.S. cities recover from disasters, evolving trends in disaster philanthropy, the public health response to Hurricane Irene, and a Federal Emergency Management Agency–funded "community tabletop" that focused on how well school systems can prepare for disasters. From 2007 to 2010, Dr. Abramson served as an associate editor of the American Medical Association peer-reviewed journal *Disaster Medicine and Public Health Preparedness*. Prior to entering the field of public health in 1990, Dr. Abramson worked for a decade as a national magazine journalist. He has written for *Rolling Stone*, *Esquire*, *Outside*, and the *San Francisco*

Examiner, among other publications. A former paramedic, Dr. Abramson holds a doctorate in sociomedical sciences with a specialization in political science and a master of public health degree, both from Columbia University.

Michael R. Anderson, M.D., FAAP (*Workshop Chair*), is vice president and chief medical officer for University Hospitals (UH) Case Medical Center and associate professor of pediatrics at Case Western Reserve School of Medicine. He specializes in pediatric critical care at UH Rainbow Babies & Children's Hospital in Cleveland, Ohio. In his role as chief medical officer, Dr. Anderson is charged with oversight of quality and patient safety; research and technology; graduate and continuing medical education; risk management; and credentialing and medical staff coordination for the 900-bed academic medical center campus, which includes the UH Seidman Cancer Center, the MacDonald Women's Hospital, and the nationally renowned Rainbow Babies and Children's Hospital. Dr. Anderson has been active at the local, state, and national levels in disaster preparedness and in 2008 was appointed by President George W. Bush to serve as vice chair to the National Commission on Children and Disasters. The 10-member commission was charged with analyzing and making recommendations to the president and Congress for the improvement of the care of children in disasters. Dr. Anderson continues to serve as a consultant to the Centers for Disease Control and Prevention and the National Disaster Medical System in the Department of Health and Human Services in Washington, DC, on pediatric disaster needs. In addition, he serves as chair of the National Children's Hospitals Disaster Task Force and has testified in front of the U.S. Senate, the Institute of Medicine, and the President's Commission on Bioethics. He is currently completing a health care executive M.B.A. program at the Kent State University School of Business.

Angie Besendorfer, Ed.L.D., serves as assistant superintendent of Joplin Schools (Missouri), a position she has held since 2007. Her areas of oversight include curriculum, instruction and accountability, special education, technology, and 21st-century learning. Since the May 2011 tornado, she has taken on roles related to the lease of temporary facilities, planning and design for four permanent buildings, and education of the Joplin public for the passage of the recent bond issue. Dr. Besendorfer served previously as superintendent for Reeds Spring School District and was elementary principal at Mill Creek Elementary in Independence and Columbian Elementary in Carthage, Missouri. She has worked as director of special services in Holden, Missouri, was assistant director of the Central Regional Professional Development Center, and was an elementary teacher in the Nevada, Missouri, district, where she was instrumental in the establishment of the Storefront School for academically at-risk students. She has been a STARR (Select Teachers As Regional Resources) program teacher and has won the Miliken Family Foundation Award. She received her bachelor's degree in education from Missouri Southern State University, her master's of science degree in elementary administration from Central Missouri State University, and her doctorate in education leadership from the University of Missouri.

Allison Blake, M.S.W., Ph.D., was appointed commissioner of the New Jersey Department of Children and Families in June 2010. As commissioner, she has emphasized an integrated and strategic approach to serving children and families in the state. To that end, Dr. Blake has focused on a community-based, family-centered approach to service delivery throughout the work of the entire department; ensured the inclusion of parent and youth voices in the department's planning and quality-improvement work; and fostered a significant expansion of partnerships with the community to help enhance child abuse prevention and family-strengthening efforts across the state. With a vision to promote sustainable growth and identify areas of improvement, as one of her first initiatives, Dr. Blake elevated the status of the Division of Child Protection and Permanency (formerly known as the Division of Youth and Family Services) office on adolescents to a department-level office with an emphasis on a more strategic approach to serving youth transitioning to adulthood. By partnering with youth, parents, stakeholders, service providers, and other state agencies to determine the current strengths of the system and the opportunities for improvement, a formal strategic plan was launched in 2011. In addition, Dr. Blake has created an internal office focused on performance management and accountability to help the department become a self-correcting, transparent organization. For almost 30 years, Dr. Blake has been working on behalf of children and families and the social workers who serve them. Prior to rejoining state service, she served as the director of the Institute for Families at the Rutgers School of Social Work, where she oversaw a portfolio of grants and contracts aimed at strengthening families by building the capacity of the individuals and organizations that serve them. She also served as vice president of accreditation operations at the Council on Accreditation (COA), an international organization that develops best-practice standards for public and private organizations that provide services across the continuum of care. Her focus while at COA was on helping agencies build their capacity to improve service delivery, a focus she has carried to her vision and work as commissioner of the Department of Children and Families. Some may view Dr. Blake's professional career as a cycle with an inevitable "homecoming," as she spent 18 years at the New Jersey Division of Youth and Family Services working in various direct service and administrative positions. She later worked with the team charged with developing a blueprint for improving the capacity of the child welfare system to improve services for the state's at-risk children and families. Dr. Blake earned her B.S. in social work from University of Dayton, an M.S. in social work from Rutgers University, and a Ph.D. in social work from Fordham University.

Judy Bezon Braune, M.S., was the associate director for Children's Disaster Services (CDS) from September 2007 to December 2012. Her responsibilities included program development and expansion; supervision of staff; training, certification and deployment of volunteers; managing interagency relations; and creating partnerships to expand the capacity of the rapid response program. Before joining CDS, Ms. Bezon Braune worked as a school psychologist, implementing several programs promoting children's mental health and utilizing play therapy techniques with at-risk and emotionally disturbed children.

Kathryn Brinsfield, M.D., M.P.H., F.A.C.E.P., serves as the acting assistant secretary of health affairs and acting chief medical officer for the Department of Homeland Security's (DHS's) Office of Health Affairs (OHA). She began her service with DHS in July 2008. Previously, she served as director of the Division of Workforce Health and Medical Support within OHA. Before joining DHS, Dr. Brinsfield worked for various organizations, including Massachusetts Homeland Security, Boston Emergency Medical Services (EMS), Boston Metropolitan Medical Response System, and the del Valle Emergency Preparedness Training Institute. Dr. Brinsfield left Boston as an associate professor at the Boston University Schools of Medicine and Public Health with 13 years of experience as an attending physician at Boston City Hospital/Boston Medical Center. She graduated with honors from

Brown University and received her M.D. from Tufts School of Medicine and her M.P.H. from Boston University. She completed her residency in emergency medicine at Cook County Hospital in Chicago and her EMS fellowship at Boston EMS. She worked for Boston EMS as director of research, training, and quality improvement; medical director for special operations; and associate medical director. She chaired the American College of Emergency Physician's Disaster Committee, co-chaired the Massachusetts State Surge Committee, assisted in the creation of the Massachusetts Alternate Standards of Care Committee, and was the commander of the Massachusetts-1 Disaster Medical Assistance Team and a supervisory medical officer for the International Medical and Surgical Response Team, which responded to the September 11 attacks.

Mary Casey-Lockyer, M.H.S., B.S.N., R.N., CCRN, is currently the manager/activity lead for Disaster Health Services at the national headquarters for the American Red Cross. Her responsibilities include Disaster Health Services program development and maintenance; supporting and coordinating the Disaster Health Services volunteer response to disasters; and fostering partnerships with federal/state/local partners and nongovernmental agencies and associations. Prior to her current position, Ms. Casey-Lockyer was an active volunteer with the American Red Cross and the Palatine, Illionois, Medical Reserve Corps. As a Disaster Health Services manager/chief with the Red Cross, she has been on 11 national deployments, most recently to the Hurricane Sandy response in New York. She also served on many volunteer project committees, including the Medical Reserve Corps partnership committee that developed the Building Block document. She received federal deployment training for the Medical Reserve Corps and participated in the Medical Reserve Corps support of the 2010 Chicago marathon. From 2002 to 2011, Ms. Casey-Lockyer was the emergency preparedness and response coordinator for Northwest Community Hospital located in Arlington Heights, Illionis. She was involved in emergency planning activities at the local, regional, state, and federal levels. Ms. Casey-Lockyer earned a master's degree in homeland security with a focus on public health preparedness in 2010 from the Pennsylvania State University Hershey School of Medicine and holds a bachelor's of science in nursing degree from DePaul University. Her nursing career includes staff nursing at Rush University Hospital, critical care open-heart nursing, and administrative supervisor roles at Northwest Community hospital.

Esther Chernak, M.D., M.P.H., is the director of the Center for Public Health Readiness and Communication at the Drexel University School of Public Health and an associate professor in the department of environmental health since 2010. At Drexel, Dr. Chernak teaches and directs research and service activities in community preparedness and building public health infrastructure. She recently collaborated with the Pennsylvania Department of Health and the Pennsylvania Chapter of the American Academy of Pediatrics to complete a strategic plan for integrating community-based pediatricians into public health preparedness planning in Pennsylvania. Her current work also includes a public health risk assessment of metropolitan Philadelphia and the state of Pennsylvania, the development of a planning aid for public health emergencies for public health and health care professionals, and oversight of the National Resource Center for Advancing Emergency Preparedness for Culturally Diverse Communities (diversitypreparedness.org), a Web-based clearing-house of resources. Dr. Chernak is an infectious diseases physician with two decades of experience in public health practice at the Philadelphia Department of Public Health. She has held a variety of positions there since 1991, including clinical director of HIV services and public health physician in the department's communicable disease control program. More recently, she served as medical director of the Acute Communicable Disease Control Program and as program manager of the Public Health Emergency Preparedness Program. Under her leadership, the department launched enhanced disease surveillance programs, a health alert network and website for public health partners, planning for pandemic influenza planning and mass prophylaxis, an outreach program to community-based organizations to reach vulnerable populations, and department-wide training in aspects of public health preparedness. In addition to her current academic position, she works as an infectious disease specialist and clinician in the health department's primary care safety net system, where she provides clinical care to individuals with HIV and guides program implementation and policy regarding infectious diseases. She was also a public health physician for the Montgomery County Health Department in Montgomery County, Pennsylvania, and served as that health department's medical director from 2000 to 2001. Her areas of interest include public health practice and preparedness, clinical infectious diseases, and initiatives that foster collaborations between public health and medical practice. She is board certified in internal medicine and infectious diseases.

Bruce Clements, M.P.H., has served as the preparedness director at the Texas Department of State Health Services since 2009. He held the equivalent position for the State of Missouri from 2005 to 2007. In this capacity, he provides leadership and oversight for public health preparedness programs and related legislative initiatives in Texas. These efforts combine the disciplines of public health, clinical medicine, emergency management, and public administration to build a state wide public health and medical emergency response infrastructure. In addition, he manages federal public health and health care system preparedness grants and provides direction for statewide preparedness activities, including preparedness planning, training, and exercises. He also serves on the Texas Commission on State Emergency Communications representing the Department of State Health Services and providing oversight of the statewide 9-1-1 and poison control programs. Mr. Clements has extensive experience in emergency response activities, including forming and managing response teams that include an environmental health team that responded to the Midwest Floods of 1993; a public health team that deployed in 1997 to Hurricane Mitch in Honduras; Missouri state responses to ice storms, floods, and tornadoes; and Texas state responses to hurricanes, wildfires, West Nile virus, and the H1N1 influenza pandemic. He also assisted in the formation of the Missouri Task Force 1, Urban Search and Rescue Team and the Missouri-1 Disaster Medical Assistance Team. During a 23-year career in the U.S. Air Force and Air National Guard, Mr. Clements served as a disaster preparedness specialist responding to a wide range of emergency situations and as a public health officer. He received a master's of public health degree from Saint Louis University in St. Louis, Missouri, and served as the associate director of the Saint Louis University Institute for Biosecurity from 2000 to 2005. The institute developed preparedness courses and multimedia education and reference materials on bioterrorism and emerging infections; planned and coordinated research initiatives to better identify and define preparedness information and training needs of health care and public health workers; and developed an online master of science in biosecurity degree program. He has current adjunct instructor appointments at the Texas A&M Health Sciences Center, School of Rural Public Health, Department of Health Policy & Management, and the University of North Texas Health Science Center, School of Public Health, Department of Environmental and Occupational Health. He has published a variety of articles on preparedness, contributed book chapters, and authored a textbook on disasters and public health. He has also lectured extensively on preparedness topics for more than 20 years.

Richard Devylder is the nation's senior advisor for accessible transportation at the U.S. Department of Transportation, appointed in July 2010 by President Obama. Mr. Devylder advises the department's efforts to develop and execute effective policy strategies to ensure that all modes of transportation are accessible and integrated to meet the diverse functional needs of the public. Mr. Devylder served as special advisor to the secretary of the California Emergency Management Agency from January 2008 to June 2010, focusing on the access and functional needs of people with disabilities in disasters. Mr. Devylder provided guidance in reviewing and reshaping emergency management systems, policies, and practices in communicating, evacuating, and sheltering Californians with disabilities. As deputy director for the California Department of Rehabilitation from August 2003 to January 2008, Mr. Devylder was responsible for the oversight of four departmental divisions. From 2001 to 2003, he served as chairman of the State Independent Living Council and as the executive director of the Dayle McIntosh Center from September 2000 to August 2003.

Dan Dodgen, Ph.D., is the director for At-Risk Individuals, Behavioral Health, and Community Resilience in the Office of the Assistant Secretary for Preparedness and Response at the U.S. Department of Health and Human Services (HHS). His office focuses on ensuring that at-risk individuals, behavioral health, and community resilience are integrated into federal public health and medical preparedness and response activities. Before joining HHS, Dr. Dodgen served as special assistant to the CEO and senior legislative and federal affairs officer at the American Psychological Association (APA). Before joining APA, Dr. Dodgen was a fellow with the U.S. House of Representatives Committee on Education. He has served on multiple federal advisory groups and authored numerous articles and book chapters on psychology and public policy. He received the APA 2005 Early Career Award for Contribution to Psychology in the Public Interest and was elected a fellow of APA in 2012. He is a licensed clinical psychologist in the District of Columbia.

George Foltin, M.D., is currently the director of the Center for Pediatric Emergency Medicine at Maimonides Infant and Children's Hospital, where he is an associate professor of pediatrics and emergency medicine at the New York University School of Medicine, and serves as the vice chair of the department of pediatrics. He is board certified in pediatrics, emergency medicine, and pediatric emergency medicine. Among his numerous committee activities, he is the chairperson of the American Academy of Pediatrics District II Committee on Emergency Medical Services for Children (EMSC), chairperson of the New York City (NYC) Task Force on Terrorism Preparedness for Children and, founding president of the New York Society for Pediatric Emergency Medicine. Since 1985, Dr. Foltin has published extensively in the field of emergency medical services for children and serves as a consultant to the New York City and New York State departments of health, as well as to federal programs such as the Maternal and Child Health Bureau and the National Highway Traffic Safety Administration. Most recently, Dr. Foltin has worked with the New York City Department of Health and Mental Hygiene (DOHMH) to develop a New York Pediatric Disaster Coalition. Previous collaborative efforts with DOHMH have included a Pediatric Blast Tabletop Disaster Exercise and a Pediatric Disaster Preparedness Toolkit for the General Hospital; and, with the national EMSC program, a similar toolkit for the prehospital community. Dr. Foltin has been and continues to be principal investigator for many federally funded grants, including a project to develop the Pediatric Terrorism and Disaster Preparedness Resource in partnership with the American Academy of Pediatrics; the Pediatric Out-of-Hospital Cardiac and Respiratory Arrest Study in NYC; a project to develop the basic and paramedic versions of the TRIPP (Teaching Resource for Instructors in Prehospital Pediatrics); and, as co-investigator, the EMSC Research Network Development Demonstration Project and the EMSC Model Pediatric Component for State Disaster Plans Project.

Patricia Frost, M.S., R.N., PNP, is the director of emergency medical services (EMS) for Contra Costa County, supporting the coordination and oversight of the EMS system serving 1.1 million people with more than 75,000 calls per year and more than 55,000 transports. She also serves as co-chair of the California Coalition for Neonatal/Pediatric Disaster Preparedness, linking novice to expert to support local disaster preparedness for infants and children. Ms. Frost is an experienced clinician and program and project manager with more than 30 years of pediatric and neonatal critical care and ambulatory experience in a variety of roles, including faculty positions at major universities, medical relief work in Ecuador and Vietnam, staff development, patient care, and advanced practice nursing. She has expertise in creating, developing, and managing programs supporting implementation of standards of care in communities, including pediatric life-support training, patient safety, quality improvement, ST Elevation Myocardial Infarction (STEMI) System Development, and STROKE systems. Among her goals is to fully integrate EMS with the health care system of Contra Costa County. Her specialties include EMS administration, program development, coalition building, pediatric emergency care, prehospital and pediatric health care provider education and training, emergency preparedness, prehospital quality improvement and safety, pediatric disaster and surge preparedness, and STEMI and STROKE system development.

Peter Gudaitis, M.Div., is president of the National Disaster Interfaiths Network—a 501(c)(3) nonprofit that provides consulting, speakers, research, and training to disaster human services and faith-based initiatives to faith communities, faith-based organizations, community-based organizations, colleges/universities, foundations, and government agencies who seek to engage and enhance the mitigation, readiness, response, and recovery capacity of faith communities and government partnerships with whole communities. He also lectures and offers trainings nationally and internationally on religious competency and building sustainable faith-based partnerships as well as disaster readiness, response, and recovery services best practices. From 2003 to 2009, Mr. Gudaitis was the executive director and CEO of New York Disaster Interfaith Services (NYDIS) and currently serves on the board of directors and as its chief response officer. NYDIS is a 501(c)(3) federation of judicatories, faith-based human service providers, and charitable organizations that work in partnership to provide disaster readiness, response, and recovery services for New York City hazards (including 9/11 response). NYDIS collaborates with local, state, and national agencies involved in facilitating the delivery of nonsectarian spiritual care, secular disaster human services, resources, and information to religious communities, underserved victims, and impacted neighborhoods. Mr. Gudaitis has more than 25 years of experience in chaplaincy, emergency management, faith-based philanthropy, program management, and social services administration. He is a former emergency medical services (EMS) supervisor and EMS chaplain. Mr. Gudaitis holds a master of divinity degree from the General Theological Seminary of the Episcopal Church and a B.A. from Kenyon College. He participates on many local and national disaster human services and nonprofit boards and committees. Mr. Gudaitis is a research associate at the University of Southern California Center for Religion and Civic Culture and a guest lecturer and member of the Emergency & Disaster Management Masters of Public Health (MPH) Advisory Board at the Metropolitan College of New York. Most recently, he was appointed to the New York State Response Commission by Governor Andrew Cuomo.

Ashley Houston is a junior at Hurricane High School in Hurricane, Utah. She is a member of the Federal Emergency Management Agency's national youth preparedness council. As such, she is charged with promoting disaster preparedness in her community as well as others, specifically focusing on youth preparedness. Ms. Houston is a Hugh O'Brian Youth alumnus as well as a Leadership Academy graduate, through which she has learned to be a leader and an effective member of society. Ms. Houston is a member of the Teen Community Emergency Response Team and also has completed the training as a Community Emergency Response Team trainer. In addition, she is a member of Hurricane's National Honor Society and is currently secretary for her school's Health Occupation Students of America. Her most recent accomplishment is the completion of a Teen Community Emergency Response Team course at her high school.

Richard Hunt, M.D., FACEP, serves as senior medical advisor for the National Healthcare Preparedness Programs in the Office of the Assistant Secretary for Preparedness and Response, U.S. Department of Health and Human Services, and as adjunct professor of emergency medicine at Emory University School of Medicine. Prior to serving in his current position, Dr. Hunt was a distinguished consultant and director of the Division of Injury Response at the National Center for Injury Prevention Control at the Centers for Disease Control and Prevention (CDC). While at CDC, he led the development of medical preparedness and response initiatives for terrorist bombings, including the guidance "In a Moment's Notice: Surge Capacity for Terrorist Bombings, and the Tale of Our Cities" conference series. He oversaw the development of CDC's guidances on "National Guidelines for Field Triage of Injured Patients"; the "Acute Injury Care Research Agenda"; and "Advanced Automatic Collision Notification and Triage of the Injured Patient." He was CDC's representative to the Federal Interagency Committee on emergency medical services (EMS). In collaboration with the World Health Organization, Dr. Hunt led CDC's work to develop and implement trauma systems in low- and middle-income countries. Prior to his work at CDC, he served as professor and chair of the department of emergency medicine at the State University of New York Upstate Medical University in Syracuse. In the field of critical care transport, Dr. Hunt was medical director of EastCare at East Carolina University School of Medicine and vice chair of the Commission on Accreditation of Medical Transport Systems. With the American College of Emergency Physicians (ACEP), he served as chair of the Trauma Care and Injury Control Committee and for 10 years was liaison from ACEP to the American College of Surgeons' Committee on Trauma. He is the founding president of Advocates for EMS and is a past president of the National Association of EMS Physicians.

Amy Knight, M.H.A., is the senior vice president of the Children's Hospital Association, representing more than 220 hospital organizations and programs dedicated to improving child health through innovation in care, education, and research. The association is the result of the 2011 merger between the former National Association of Children's Hospitals and Related Institutions, the National Association of Children's Hospitals, and Child Health Corporation of America and comprises more than 200 staff advancing public policy, business performance improvement, quality, and advocacy with its member hospitals. Ms. Knight's specific responsibilities include oversight of marketing, policy, and corporate communications, public relations, governance, member relations, and education. The association currently has offices in Alexandria, Virginia, and Overland Park, Kansas. Ms. Knight joined the association in November 2011. She was previously a partner in the health care practice at Kurt Salmon, a global consulting firm. In this capacity, she also served as the director of Children's Hospital Services. As a strategic advisor to children's hospitals and academic medical centers across the nation, she understands their strategic and operating issues in the evolving legislative, payor, and regulatory environments. She routinely led engagements with hospital executive teams and boards to position their enterprises for success in their local, regional, and national markets. Ms. Knight has a master's of health administration degree from Washington University's School of Medicine in St. Louis and a bachelor of arts degree in history from the University of Texas at Austin.

Evelyn Lyons, B.S.N., M.P.H., is the manager and co–principal investigator of the Illinois Emergency Medical Services for Children (EMSC) program within the Division of EMS & Highway Safety, Illinois Department of Public Health. She has coordinated the Illinois EMSC program since 1994. In this role, her responsibilities involve developing and implementing pediatric emergency care and disaster preparedness initiatives within the state of Illinois, as well as coordinating several data projects that are conducted in conjunction with the Illinois Department of Transportation. Her background includes public health, grants management, and quality improvement as well as more than 30 years of experience in emergency nursing and emergency medical services. She received a bachelor of science in nursing degree from St. Xavier University, Chicago, Illinois, in 1977 and a master's of public health degree from Benedictine University, Lisle, Illinois, in 1998.

Gregg Margolis, Ph.D., NREMT-P, is the director of the Division of Healthcare Systems and Heath Policy for the Office of the Assistant Secretary of Preparedness and Response at the U.S. Department of Health and Human Services. He leads a team of policy experts in formulating, analyzing, and implementing policies to build strong, integrated, and resilient health systems that are prepared to respond to and recover from disasters and public health emergencies. Prior to his federal service, Dr. Margolis was the associate director of the National Registry of Emergency Medical Technicians, a nonprofit organization that serves as the national certification agency for almost 300,000 emergency medical services professionals. Dr. Margolis has held leadership positions and faculty appointments at the George Washington University, the University of Pittsburgh, and the Center for Emergency Medicine of Western Pennsylvania. In 2009-2010, Dr. Margolis was the first paramedic to be awarded a Robert Wood Johnson Foundation Health Policy Fellowship, through which he served in the Office of Senator John D. Rockefeller.

Ann Masten, Ph.D., LP, is the Irving B. Harris Professor of Child Development and Distinguished McKnight University Professor in the Institute of Child Development at the University of Minnesota. She completed her Ph.D. in psychology at the University of Minnesota and her clinical psychology internship at the University of California, Los Angeles. Her research focuses on understanding processes that promote competence and resilience in the context of adversity and trauma. She directs the Project Competence studies of risk and resilience, including studies of normative populations and individuals exposed to war, natural disaster, poverty, homelessness, and migration. Dr. Masten is currently a member of the Board on Children, Youth, and Families (BCYF), Institute of Medicine (IOM)/National Research Council, the U.S. National Committee of Psychology, and the Governing Council of the Society for Research in Child Development (as past president). She served on the BCYF Committee on the Impact of Mobility and Change on the Lives of Young Children, Schools, and Neighborhoods and currently serves on the collaborative IOM planning committee for Investing in Young Children Globally and the planning group for the workshop on Medical and Public Health Disaster and Preparedness Response for Children and Families. She has published widely on topics related to resilience in human development, including reviews on children and families exposed to disaster, war, and terrorism. She has received numerous honors, most recently the 2014 Urie Bronfenbrenner Award for Lifetime Contribution to Developmental Psychology in the Service of Science and Society from the American Psychological Association.

Janice Molnar, Ph.D., is deputy commissioner of the Division of Child Care Services in the New York State Office of Children and Family Services (OCFS). OCFS provides oversight and monitoring of more than 21,000 regulated child care providers and another 47,000 legally exempt providers in New York State. Throughout her 30-year career, which has included work in the public and nonprofit sectors, Dr. Molnar has concentrated on program and policy issues affecting children, youth, and families. Trained as a developmental psychologist, she has a background in research and evaluation and has experience in organizational development and organizational learning, cross-sector planning and process facilitation, and evaluation and assessment of educational and human service activities both in the United States and internationally. She earned a B.A. from Northwestern University and holds a Ph.D. from Cornell University, where her dissertation focused on the impacts of different kinds of child care arrangements on selected indicators of child development.

Scott Needle, M.D., FAAP, is a community pediatrician in Naples, Florida, and a member of the American Academy of Pediatrics's (AAP's) Disaster Preparedness Advisory Council. His personal and professional experiences on the Mississippi Gulf Coast after Hurricane Katrina have led to national attention regarding disaster-related children's health issues, pediatric private practice, disaster preparedness, and health problems related to Federal Emergency Management Agency trailers. He is the author of "A Disaster Preparedness Plan for Pediatricians," which was developed as an interactive online tool for the AAP's website. His article "Private Practice After Hurricane Katrina: A Proposal for Recovery" was published in the October 2008 issue of *Pediatrics*, followed by "The Art of the Possible: Looking Back and Ahead Five Years After Landfall" in the August 2011 *Supplement to Pediatrics*. In April 2011 he represented Florida at the AAP–Centers for Disease Control and Prevention meeting Enhancing Pediatric Partnerships to Promote Pandemic Preparedness, and was co-author on the related commentary "Improving Pediatric Preparedness Performance Through Strategic Partnerships" (published in June 2012 in *Disaster Medicine and Public Health Preparedness*). Since 2012, he has been a consultant to the Pennsylvania Chapter of the AAP for the Philadelphia-area Community Preparedness Project, in cooperation with the Drexel University School of Public Health and the Pennsylvania Department of Health. This project seeks to bring primary care pediatricians and health departments together for disaster preparedness, response, and communications. Dr. Needle has also contributed to work on community resilience, pediatric medical countermeasures, pediatric disaster education, and anthrax guidelines. He received his M.D. degree from the Johns Hopkins University School of Medicine in Baltimore, Maryland, and completed his pediatric internship and residency at New England Medical Center/Tufts University in Boston, Massachusetts.

Georgina Peacock, M.D., is a medical officer and developmental-behavioral pediatrician at the Centers for Disease Control and Prevention's (CDC's) National Center on Birth Defects and Developmental Disabilities. She is currently working with CDC's Office of Public Health Preparedness and Response on an initiative to enhance public health disaster preparedness and response for children. In addition, Dr. Peacock continues to see patients in a developmental clinic at the Good Samaritan Health Center and is an adjunct professor with the Georgia State Center for Leadership in Disability and Georgia State Leadership Education in Neurodevelopmental & Related Disabilities (LEND) program. Dr. Peacock received her doctor of medicine and master of public health degrees from the University of Kansas. She completed her pediatric residency training at the University of Kansas. She is also a former LEND trainee who completed her developmental-behavioral pediatrics fellowship at the Developmental Disabilities Center at the University of Kansas Medical Center. She initially joined CDC as an Association for University Centers on Disabilities fellow.

Irwin Redlener, M.D., is the director of the National Center for Disaster Preparedness at the Columbia University Mailman School of Public Health, which works to understand and improve the nation's capacity to prepare for, respond to, and recover from disasters. He is a nationally recognized expert on disaster preparedness policies, pandemic influenza, the threat of terrorism in the United States, the impact and consequences of major natural disasters, and related issues. Following Hurricane Sandy, Dr. Redlener was appointed by Governor Andrew Cuomo to co-chair the New York State Ready Commission, and he also recently served as 1 of the 10 members of the congressionally established National Commission on Children and Disasters. He is the author of *Americans at Risk: Why We Are Not Prepared for Megadisasters and What We Can Do Now*, published in August 2006 by Alfred A. Knopf, Inc. Dr. Redlener is also president and co-founder, with Paul Simon, of the Children's Health Fund, a philanthropic initiative created to develop health care programs in 25 of the nation's most medically underserved urban and rural communities. Under his leadership, the Children's Health Fund has grown to become a national network of more than 50 mobile and fixed-site pediatric clinics providing more than 250,000 health care encounters each year. Dr. Redlener received his M.D. from the University of Miami School of Medicine and his pediatric training at Babies Hospital of the Columbia-Presbyterian Medical Center in New York City, the University of Colorado Medical Center, and the University of Miami-Jackson Memorial Hospital in Miami. He holds honorary doctoral degrees from Hunter College of the City University of New York and Hofstra University, among numerous other awards and honors.

Marcie Roth is director of the Office of Disability Integration and Coordination of the U.S. Department of Homeland Security, Federal Emergency Management Agency (FEMA), a position to which she was appointed by President Obama in 2009. Ms. Roth serves as senior advisor to Administrator Fugate and as director of the FEMA Office of Disability Integration and Coordination, supporting implementation of objectives toward achieving the President's National Preparedness Goal and leading the national transformation toward integrating the access and functional needs of children and adults with disabilities in all aspects of whole-community emergency preparedness and disaster response, recovery, and mitigation. Ms. Roth joined FEMA after serving for more than 20 years in senior leadership positions with national and international disability policy organizations. She led national private-sector response to the additional needs of survivors with disabilities during and after Hurricanes Katrina and Rita, and she was commended by the White House for her efforts on behalf of New Yorkers with disabilities in the aftermath of the 2001 terrorist attacks. She has been deployed to New York since early November as a member of the Hurricane Sandy Joint Field Office Command Staff, where she manages a team of 15 disability integration advisors.

Andrew Rucks, Ph.D., is professor in the department of health care organization and policy at the University of Alabama at Birmingham School of Public Health. He has more than 30 years of academic and business experience. He has authored 2 books, 9 computer programming aids, and more than 75 articles and cases that have appeared in *Public Health Reports*, *Journal of Homeland Security and Emergency Preparedness*, *Long Range Planning*, *Journal of Systems Management*, *Business Horizons*, *Maternal and Child Health Journal*, *International Journal of Mass Emergencies and Disasters*, and others. Dr. Rucks works extensively with state and local health departments. His focus is on developing a regional pediatric disaster surge network for response to disasters affecting children, continuity of operations planning, strategic planning, budgeting, preparedness exercises and drills, and process optimization. Dr. Rucks also serves as the executive director of the survey research unit of the University of Alabama at Birmingham and as executive director of the Southeastern Regional Pediatric Disaster Surge Network. His academic teaching focuses on finance, leadership, and management.

David Schonfeld, M.D., FAAP, is a developmental-behavioral pediatrician and the pediatrician-in-chief and director of the National Center for School Crisis and Bereavement at St. Christopher's Hospital for Children and chair of the department of pediatrics at Drexel University College of Medicine. He is a member the American Academy of Pediatrics Disaster Preparedness Advisory Council and the Sandy

Hook Commission in Conneticut, and served as a commissioner for the National Commission on Children and Disasters. Dr. Schonfeld established the School Crisis Response Program in 1991 at Yale University School of Medicine, which provided training to tens of thousands of school-related personnel in school systems throughout the country and abroad and provided technical assistance in hundreds of school crisis events. He consulted for the New York City (NYC) Department of Education to help optimize the infrastructure within the system for crisis preparedness and response and to provide training to and technical assistance in the aftermath of the events of September 11, 2001, which included the training of approximately 1,000 district and school-level crisis teams. In 2005, Dr. Schonfeld was awarded funding by the September 11th Children's Fund and the National Philanthropic Trust to establish a National Center for School Crisis and Bereavement (NCSCB); additional funding from the New York Life Foundation provides partial support for ongoing services. The goal of the NCSCB is to promote an appreciation of the role schools can serve to support students, staff, and families at times of crisis and loss; to collaborate with organizations and agencies to further this goal; and to serve as a resource for information, training materials, consultation, and technical assistance. Dr. Schonfeld has provided consultation and training on school crises and pediatric bereavement in the aftermath of a number of school crisis events and disasters in the United States and abroad, including school and community shootings in Newtown, Connecticut, Aurora, Colorado, and Chardon, Ohio; flooding from Hurricanes Sandy in NYC and New Jersey, Katrina in New Orleans, Louisiana, and Ike in Galveston, Texas; tornadoes in Joplin, Missouri, and Alabama; and the 2008 earthquake in Sichuan, China.

Merritt Schreiber, Ph.D., is associate clinical professor and director, psychological programs, in the Center for Disaster Medicine, University of California, Irvine, School of Medicine. Dr. Schreiber is involved in the development of best-practice models bridging disaster medical, mental, and public health in mass casualty events. Dr. Schreiber has developed the PsySTART Rapid Mental Health Triage and Incident Management System for use in 88 hospitals and 33 community clinics in Los Angeles County, the District of Columbia, in statewide implementation in Minnesota, and nationally with American Red Cross disaster mental health. He is the originator of a novel psychological first aid program for children, parents, teachers, and family members called

"Listen, Protect, and Connect" featured on the U.S. Department of Homeland Security's Ready.gov/kids website. Dr. Schreiber is also the primary developer of "Anticipate, Plan, and Deter," a disaster responder resilience system being developed for LA County Emergency Medical personnel and other federal response assets. Dr. Schreiber is currently the mental health team lead for National Disaster Medical System/Disaster Medical Assistance System CA-1 and state disaster mental health advisor for the American Red Cross for Southern California. Dr. Schreiber is a member of the California Disaster Mental Health Coalition serving as an expert in children's issues in disasters. Dr. Schreiber was deployed to the Sandy Hook school shooting as the Department of Health and Human Services (HHS) Behavioral Health LNO in Newtown, Connecticut, and to the Boston Marathon bombing for the HHS/National Disaster Medical System. Dr. Schreiber was reserve captain, U.S. Public Health Service (USPHS), and served on detached service to the Office of the Command Surgeon, NORAD-USNORTHCOM, U.S. Department of Defense (DoD), from 2008 to 2010. In this role, Dr. Schreiber supported the NORTHCOM SG in the development of force mental health protection and resilience strategies and response to mental health issues in catastrophic medical events for the DoD Defense Support to Civilian Authority mission. Dr. Schreiber received the Joint Meritorious Service Medal from U.S. Northern Command in 2009 for these efforts. For the USPHS, Dr. Schreiber was activated in support of the CDC Emergency Operations Center in response to the Southeast Asian Tsunami and Hurricane Katrina. Dr. Schreiber has developed the first concept of operations (CONOPS) for LA County Department of Mental Heatlh, Seattle and King County Public Health and the first National Children's Disaster Mental Health Concept of Operations with the National Child Traumatic Stress Network's Terrorism Disaster Center at the University of Oklahoma Health Sciences Center. Dr. Schreiber currently serves on the National Academies of Science Institute of Medicine Committee on Crisis Standards of Care. Dr. Schreiber received the California Psychological Association Distinguished Humanitarian Contribution Award and a presidential citation from the American Psychological Association for his work related to 9/11. For his federal service, Dr. Schreiber received the Crisis Response Award, Outstanding Unit Citation, and Special Commendation from the U.S. Surgeon General for his development of USPHS response team disaster training.

Linda K. Smith is the deputy assistant secretary and interdepartmental liaison for early childhood development for the Administration for Children and Families (ACF) at the U.S. Department of Health and Human Services. In this role, she provides overall policy coordination for the Head Start and Early Head Start Program and the Child Care and Development Fund, as well as serving as the liaison to the U.S. Department of Education and other federal agencies. Her office serves as a focal point for early childhood policy at the federal level. Ms. Smith previously served as the executive director for the National Association of Child Care Resource and Referral Agencies (NACCRRA), where she represented more than 650 community-based agencies concerned with the care of children in their earliest years. Ms. Smith led the organization through significant growth and transformation—she was the driving force behind NACCRRA's national policy agenda and strategic plan to improve the quality of child care nationwide. Key components of NACCRRA's advocacy efforts included strengthening child care licensing and oversight, requiring comprehensive background checks, and establishing minimum training requirements for all child care workers. Prior to joining NACCRRA, Ms. Smith served as a legislative fellow and professional staffer on the Senate Health, Education, Labor and Pensions Committee under the chairmanship of the late Senator Edward M. Kennedy. Prior to this work, she was the director of the Office of Family Policy for the Secretary of Defense, where she was one of the primary architects of the military's child care program. In addition, Ms. Smith has held positions with both the U.S. Army and the U.S. Air Force. Ms. Smith began her career in early childhood education on the Northern Cheyenne Reservation in her native state of Montana. She is a graduate of the University of Montana.

Robert W. Smith, M.D., M.B.A., FAAFP, is a senior medical director for the Central Region of UnitedHealthcare Clinical Services, a division of UnitedHealthcare, the nation's largest health insurer. Responsible for clinical excellence, Dr. Smith supervises a team of medical directors focused on implementing clinical innovation, improving affordability, and ensuring availability of appropriate and timely care. Dr. Smith previously served as a market medical director for UnitedHealthcare in Missouri and southern Illinois. Prior to that, he served in the department of family medicine of the University of Pittsburgh School of Medicine as vice chair for education. Clinically active until early 2008, he was on the medical staff of several University of Pittsburgh Medical Center

(UPMC) Health System facilities. UPMC is one of the largest integrated care systems in the nation. Other significant previous roles include acting chief medical officer for a start-up and licensing phase of a new Medicaid health maintenance organization in Erie, Pennsylvania; residency director of the Meadville Medical Center Family Medicine Residency in Meadville, Pennsylvania; and executive vice president of medical affairs of the Health Care Group of St. Louis, PC. A native of Los Angeles, Dr. Smith graduated from the University of Southern California with a B.A. in psychology (cum laude) and received his M.D. from the University of California, Irvine, College of Medicine. He completed his residency training while on active duty in the U.S. Navy at the Naval Regional Medical Center, Camp Pendleton, California. Dr. Smith is board certified and currently recertified by the American Board of Family Medicine and is a fellow in the American Academy of Family Physicians. He is a member of the Christian Medical Dental Association and a life member of the American College of Physician Executives. In addition, Dr. Smith completed a graduate extension certificate in executive medical management through the extension program at the Graduate School of Management at the University of California, Irvine. He also holds an M.B.A. from the Keller Graduate School of Management of DeVry University (with distinction), where he won the coveted national George P. Doherty Award for excellence. Dr. Smith served until recently on the National Advisory Board of DeVry University. He recently served on the board of directors for Juvenile Diabetes Research Foundation, St. Louis, and the Institute for Family Medicine, St. Louis, and was an active member of the Honor Guard of American Legion Post 388 in O'Fallon, Missouri. Dr. Smith's teaching, practice, and management experience includes rural and urban settings in California, Florida, Georgia, Missouri, Pennsylvania, the Republic of the Philippines, the Republic of Panama, and while deployed at sea and in Europe aboard the former U.S.S. Guam (LPH-9) as an amphibious task force (ATF) medical director (commander ATF surgeon). He has extensive experience in the public and private sector and in both for profit and not-for-profit entities.

Kathy J. Spangler, CAE, CPRP, Ph.D. (Hon.), serves as vice president, U.S. Programs for Save the Children, where she manages the domestic commitment to creating immediate and lasting change for children in need. Save the Children, U.S. Programs, is focused on improving educational outcomes for children living in poverty through early childhood development, literacy, physical activity, and nutrition. In addition, Save the Children is the preeminent organization dedicated to protecting children during emergencies and disasters and focuses on preparedness and response efforts. Previously, at America's Promise Alliance, Dr. Spangler served in a variety of executive-level positions, including chief development officer, chief operating officer, and executive vice president of partnerships and programs from 2007 to 2010. Dr. Spangler served as the founding director of national partnerships for the National Recreation and Park Association (NRPA). Dr. Spangler's 20 years of dedicated service at the NRPA created a lasting impact the field of parks and recreation in the areas of healthy lifestyles, youth development, environmental stewardship, and high-quality sports. Dr. Spangler is a recognized leader in health promotion and was responsible for writing and directing two Centers for Disease Control and Prevention cooperative agreements, two National Institutes of Health programs, and multiple grants from corporations and foundations. She served as a national spokesperson for physical activity and nutrition, working with federal agencies and Congress on environmental policy changes promoting healthy lifestyles and livable communities. Dr. Spangler received her bachelor's degree from the University of Maine at Presque Isle in 1979, was recognized as alumnus of the year in 1998, and received an honorary doctorate in 2003. She is a past president of the National Coalition for Promoting Physical Activity and has served on the executive committee for the U.S. Tennis Association.

Ginny Sprang, Ph.D., is a professor in the College of Medicine, department of psychiatry, at the University of Kentucky, and the executive director of the UK Center on Trauma and Children, a center whose mission is dedicated to the enhancement of the health and the well-being of children and their families through research, service, and dissemination of information about traumatic stress in pediatric populations. Dr. Sprang is the principal investigator of several projects funded by the Substance Abuse and Mental Health Services Administration, the Department of Homeland Security, and the Health Resources and Services Administration that examine treatment effectiveness and best practices protocols for disaster-, violence-, and trauma-exposed children and families. Dr. Sprang received her Ph.D. from the University of Texas in 1991 and served as a visiting associate professor in the department of psychiatry at the University of Colorado

Health Science Center, Irving Harris Program in Child Development and Infant Mental Health, during her sabbatical. Dr. Sprang serves as the chair of the Bioterrorism and Terrorism Disaster Special Interest Group of the International Society for Traumatic Stress Studies, has served on the steering committee for the National Child Traumatic Stress Network, and is the national co-chair of the Secondary Traumatic Stress Committee for that organization. Dr. Sprang has published extensively in the area of child traumatic stress, victimization, and post-disaster recovery of adult and pediatric populations.

Kari Tatro is the executive vice president of emergency management operations for BCFS Health and Human Services, an international system of nonprofit corporations. Ms. Tatro operates a comprehensive emergency management program for all-hazards planning, preparedness, response, and recovery operations, with specific emphasis on medical needs operations; functional needs support services; and all other health and medical emergencies. She has functioned as command staff for multiple incidents, including as incident commander of medical needs operations for Hurricanes Dolly, Gustav, and Ike. Ms. Tatro is a foremost expert on emergency planning for people with disabilities and others with access and functional needs and served as the executive manager and subject-matter expert responsible for developing the Federal Emergency Management Agency document and curriculum on integrating Functional Need Support Services (FNSS) into general population sheltering, published in 2010. Ms. Tatro provides training and consultation across the nation at conferences, symposiums, and one-on-one training for jurisdictions requesting specific assistance with interpretation of the FNSS guidelines and/or implementation. Ms. Tatro started her career as a wildland fire fighter for the U.S. Forest Service, moving to a position where she coordinated planning, mitigation, response, and recovery for local, state, and federal governments in Texas. Prior to her career with BCFS, Ms. Tatro served as a regional liaison officer with the Texas Division of Emergency Management. In this time, she assisted local and tribal governments in developing and implementing local emergency operation plans, developing and coordinating disaster exercises and securing, and coordinating state and federal response assets to support jurisdictional disasters. Ms. Tatro had an integral role in coordinating the regional state response to Hurricane Rita for 16 counties in eastern Texas, including evacuation operations for eight counties and shelter operations in eight hosting counties, sheltering a population of more than 40,000 persons.

Joyce A. Thomas, M.A., is the regional administrator for the Administration for Children and Families (ACF) in ACF Region II. The region comprises New Jersey, New York, Puerto Rico, and the U.S. Virgin Islands. In this capacity, Ms. Thomas partners with state, local, and community-based organizations and tribes within the region to promote economic independence and healthy development of children and families. Ms. Thomas provides executive leadership and direction to ensure coordination and integration of activities among Head Start, child care, foster care and adoption, child support enforcement, youth services, and Temporary Assistance to Needy Families (TANF) programs. Ms. Thomas serves as national lead regional administrator for the Office of Community Services and the Faith-Based and Neighborhood Partnership Initiatives within ACF. She is one of the founders and co-chairs of ACF's African American Healthy Marriage Initiative. Previously, Ms. Thomas served as the regional administrator for ACF's Region V, which includes Illinois, Indiana, Michigan, Minnesota, Ohio, Wisconsin, and 35 tribal nations. While Region V administrator, Ms. Thomas also led the federal regional Interagency Council on Homelessness. Under Emergency Preparedness and Response, ACF Region II partners with the Federal Emergency Management Agency, state government, grantees, and tribes to ensure coordination of essential human services programs during disasters. Ms. Thomas has played pivotal roles in coordinating on-the-ground responses to Hurricane Irene (2011) and Superstorm Sandy (2012 and continuing), the largest storm in history in the Atlantic Ocean in terms of size and the second-costliest hurricane ever to make landfall in the United States. Ms. Thomas was the recipient of the Assistant Secretary for Children and Families' 2012 Exemplary Leadership Award for her work concerning Hurricane Irene. Prior to her employment with ACF, Ms. Thomas served as the commissioner of Connecticut's Department of Social Services. As Commissioner, she implemented major changes in the child support enforcement, TANF, and Medicaid programs and played a major role in the creation of Connecticut's innovative School Readiness legislation. A graduate of the University of Northern Iowa, Ms. Thomas received a B.A. in social work and an M.A. in counseling, with a minor in Spanish.

Jeff Upperman, M.D., is an associate professor of surgery in the department of surgery at the Keck School of Medicine at the University of Southern California. He is an attending faculty surgeon, director of the trauma program, Pediatric Disaster Resource and Training Center, and program director for the Pediatric Surgery Fellowship Program at Children's Hospital Los Angeles. Dr. Upperman graduated from Stanford University in 1987 with a bachelor's degree in human biology and a master's degree in sociology. He earned his medical degree and completed his surgical residency at New Jersey Medical School. Dr. Upperman's research interests include trauma, injury prevention, sepsis, inflammation, and disaster preparedness. Dr. Upperman practices at Children's Hospital Los Angeles and in the San Fernando Valley.

Lieutenant Commander Jonathan White, Ph.D., LCSW-C, is the deputy director of the Office of Human Services Emergency Preparedness and Response at the U.S. Department of Health and Human Services' Administration for Children and Families. He is a commissioned officer in the U.S. Public Health Service and a licensed clinical social worker. He holds an M.S.W. in clinical and macro social work from the Catholic University of America, a Ph.D. in American literature from George Washington University, a licensed certified social worker–clinical license, and social work supervisor certification from the State of Maryland, and is a board-certified diplomate in clinical social work. He has worked previously as a hospital social worker specializing in work with advanced oncology patients, disaster mental health responder, college English professor, and labor union campaign staffer.

John Wible, J.D., is general counsel (retired), Alabama Department of Public Health (ADPH), and currently adjunct professor of public health law at the University of Alabama School of Law. At ADPH, he served as assistant attorney general; as chief legal officer to the department; and as advisor to the state health officer, State Board of Health, and state-level and county-level public health agencies. He managed ADPH's grants and contracts and supervised all litigation, legislation, and rule-making procedures. He served as bioterrorism counsel and Health Insurance Portability and Accountability Act privacy officer and chaired ADPH's institutional review board and compliance committee. He taught Continuing Legal Education courses on public health–related subjects and taught seminars for the South Central Center for Public Health, University of South Alabama, Tulane University School of Public Health and Tropical Medicine, and University of Alabama at Birmingham School of Public Health. He also serves as a visiting lecturer, University of South Alabama, School of Medicine, and as the State Mortuary Response Team's Family Assistance Center executive director. At Gateway Baptist Church in Montgomery, Alabama, he serves as volunteer worship coordinator; Sunday School teacher; principal, Gateway Academy and tutoring program; liaison to Korean Church congregation; teacher, English as a second language; and teacher, American history. He has taken missions trips to Brazil, Canada, India, and various U.S. cities.

Patricia Wright, Ph.D., M.P.H., has a passion for education and advocacy and has dedicated her career to ensuring that individuals with autism are fully included in society. Her personal mission is to offer support that makes it possible for people with autism lead meaningful, happy, and productive lives. As Easter Seals' national director of autism services, Dr. Wright leads autism programs for Easter Seals, one of the nation's largest providers of services for individuals with autism across the life span. Dr. Wright's expertise as an educator and board-certified behavior analyst inform her individualized approach to creating effective treatment plans. She knows that early diagnosis and intervention offer the best outcomes but also is a proponent of appropriate treatment for anyone with autism at any age. Everyone has the ability to learn and develop skills. She is a member of the Organization for Autism Research's scientific council and has served on the executive committee for the Friends of the Centers for Disease Control and Prevention's National Center for Birth Defects and Developmental Disabilities. Dr. Wright earned her Ph.D. in education from the University of Hawaii in 2006. She also has an M.P.H. from the University of Hawaii and a master's degree in special education from San Francisco State University.

F

Resource List: Tools for Planning for Children and Families

NOTE: This list is not comprehensive, but is meant to be a compilation of tools and resources highlighted by speakers during the workshop and mentioned throughout the summary.

PSYCHOLOGICAL FIRST AID/BEHAVIORAL TRAINING	
Department of Health and Human Services (HHS) Disaster Behavioral Health Concept of Operations	http://www.phe.gov/Preparedness/planning/abc/Documents/dbh-conops.pdf
National Child Traumatic Stress Network: 6 hour interactive Psychological Aid Online Training	http://learn.nctsn.org/course/category.php?id=11
National Child Traumatic Stress Network: *Psychological First Aid Field Operations Guide*	http://www.nctsn.org/content/psychological-first-aid
Web-based learning: Trauma-Focused Cognitive Behavioral Therapy	http://tfcbt.musc.edu

PLANNING TOOLS AND RESOURCES	
Administration for Children and Families/HHS: Early Childhood Disaster Related Resources	http://www.acf.hhs.gov/programs/ohsepr/early-childhood
American Academy of Pediatrics	http://www.aap.org/en-us/advocacy-and-policy/aap-health-initiatives/Children-and-Disasters/Documents/Ped PreparednessKit.pdf
Contra Costa County Pedi/Neo Disaster and Medical Surge Plan and Resources	http://cchealth.org/ems/emsc-disaster-prepare.php
New York City (NYC) Pediatric Disaster	http://cpem.med.nyu.edu/teaching

Coalition: Planning, Management, and Provision of Out-of-Hospital Care	materials/pediatric-disaster-preparedness
Office of the Assistant Secretary for Preparedness and Response (ASPR) June 2013 Technical Assistance Webinar and Resources	http://www.phe.gov/Preparednes/planning/abc/Pages/webinar-resources-130620.aspx
Pediatric Preparedness Resource Catalog–Illinois Department of Public Health	http://www.luhs.org/depts/emsc/disaster_preparedness/PedPrepareResourceDev_2009web_V2.pdf
PEDIATRIC TRAINING FOR HEALTH PROFESSIONALS	
Gamification of Learning via LA Children's Hospital: Disaster Olympix Video	http://www.youtube.com/watch?v=sZVgdRj-bCc
Gamification of Learning via LA Children's Hospital: Surge World	http://lachildrenshospital.net/SurgeWorld
NYC Pediatric Disaster Coalition: Hospital guidelines for Pediatric Preparedness and Tabletop Exercise Toolkit	http://www.nyc.gov/html/doh/html/em/emergency-ped.shtml
Pediatric Fundamental Critical Care Support (PFCCS) Course	http://www.sccm.org/Fundamentals/PFCCS/Pages/default.aspx
Planning and Response to a Pandemic Event Supporting Children and Families	http://www.cecentral.com/node/433
Tracking and Reuniting Children in Disasters	http://ncdmph.usuhs.edu/KnowledgeLearning/2012-Learning1.htm
University of New Mexico Pediatric Emergency Training Online Education Program	http://hsc.unm.edu/emermed/PED/education/onlineEd.shtml
DEPARTMENT OF CHILDREN AND FAMILIES/CHILD CARE	
Head Start Emergency Preparedness Manual	http://eclkc.ohs.acf.hhs.gov/hslc/tta-system/health/ep
Long-Term Recovery Plan to Support Children and Families	http://www.state.nj.us/dcf/home/HurricaneSandyRecoveryPlan.pdf
Protecting Children in Child Care During Emergencies–Save the Children and Child Care Aware	http://www.naccrra.org/sites/default/files/publications/naccrra_publications/2012/protectingchildreninchildcareemergencies.pdf
Videos for Child Care Providers in Emergency Scenarios	http://www.ecetp.pdp.albany.edu/videolibrary.shtm#emergencyvids

COMMUNICATION TOOLS/WORKING WITH PEOPLE WITH DISABILITIES	
Communication Toolkit for Public Health Emergencies Affecting Children	https://www.portal.state.pa.us/portal/server.pt/document/1337530/final_aap_toolkit_5_2_13_pdf
Emergency Communication for People with Complex Communication Needs	http://aac-rerc.psu.edu/index.php/pages/show/id/4
Planning and Training Resources for Working with People with Disabilities	http://www.ohsu.edu/xd/research/centers-institutes/institute-on-development-and-disability/public-health-programs/oodh-emergency-preparedness.cfm
University of Vermont Self-Help Emergency Toolkit	http://www.uvm.edu/~cdci/gmep/GrnMtnGuideforEmergPlan_forprint.pdf
RELIGIOUS ORGANIZATION TIP SHEETS	
Training, Resources and Tip Sheets for Religious Leaders and Faith Community Partners to Build "Ready Congregations"	http://www.n-din.org

G

The Science and Practice of Resilience Interventions for Children Exposed to Disasters

David Abramson, Ph.D., Columbia University
Kallin Brooks, J.D., Columbia University
Lori Peek, Ph.D., Colorado State University

A white paper prepared for the June 10-11, 2013, workshop on Disaster Preparedness, Response, and Recovery Considerations for Children and Families, hosted by the Institute of Medicine's (IOM's) Forum on Medical and Public Health Preparedness for Catastrophic Events. The authors are responsible for the content of this article, which does not necessarily represent the views of the IOM.

PROLOGUE

The post-Katrina trailer park where we met "M" was markedly different from the many others that had sprung up in the weeks and months following the devastating 2005 hurricane. Rather than being situated in a dusty field, surrounded by chain-link fencing, this trailer park was in a forested glen. The houses were well-kept, single-wide mobile homes, arranged in a horseshoe shape around a grassy field, rather than the smaller travel trailers arranged in endless rows common to other trailer parks. Our research team of interviewers pulled up to this trailer park mid-afternoon just as the school bus arrived. Twenty to 30 schoolchildren emptied from the bus and went running across the field to their homes. Many knew each other from their old New Orleans neighborhood in the Lower Ninth Ward. The residents were mainly working-class and working-poor residents who had been displaced from their homes, and represented a mix of homeowners and renters living in this Federal Emergency Management Agency (FEMA)-subsidized emergency housing.

Our team of 15 researchers fanned out across the trailer park to recruit the mobile home residents to our Gulf Coast Child and Family Health Study. This was the baseline survey for what would ultimately be a 5-year longitudinal cohort study of 1,079 randomly sampled households in Louisiana and Mississippi. The interviews generally took about 45 minutes. One of the interviewers emerged from a home after 2 hours with the resident. She was visibly moved as she recounted the woman's story.

"M" was in her late 40s, a mother of 2 children, 1 high-school-aged, the other an adult. During the hurricane, "M" was separated from her husband and daughters, because she had been required to report to the health care facility where she worked and ended up evacuating with the patients. For almost a week, the family did not know of one another's fate, or even whether they had survived the storm. They ended up reunited at a Texas shelter, and during the succeeding 6 months leading up to our interview, they moved 7 times, across multiple states. As "M" described her journey to our interviewer, she pulled out a scrapbook. It was filled with pictures—of her destroyed home in New Orleans, and then of every place where she and the family had stayed since the hurricane. They had moved from shelter to shelter, to hotels and motels, to crowded homes where they doubled up with friends, and ultimately to this trailer park. Her husband drove their teenaged daughter back and forth to her old New Orleans high school daily, commuting up to 4 hours in an effort to maintain this stability in their daughter's life. The snapshots in the scrapbook chronicled this story. "Whenever my girls face something difficult in their lives, I want them to be able to pull this scrapbook out," "M" told our interviewer. "I want them to see where they've been, the challenges they've faced. This is their strength. There isn't anything they can't handle."

Our research team re-interviewed "M" three more times in the subsequent 5 years. Two years after the hurricane, the team found her living in a travel trailer in the front yard of her New Orleans home as she supervised its reconstruction. By the last round of interviewing, she and her family had moved back in to their home, and her daughter had graduated from high school and was attending college. It appeared that the family had regained its pre-hurricane stability despite almost 5 years of enormously difficult economic and social hardships.

As a tale of resilience, "M"'s story reflects so many of the characteristics and attributes identified by researchers. Despite exposure to extreme adversity, "M"'s daughter maintained critical academic routines, was encouraged by her parents to develop her cognitive skills, was living in a supportive and nurturing household with a mother who actively promoted her daughter's sense of self-efficacy and hope for the future (embodied by a tangible tool—the scrapbook—to reinforce the message). "M" herself was a woman who personified "hardiness" and whose personal outlook was dominated by her faith, good humor, and unshakable optimism. At a larger level, her daughter's resilience was further bolstered by the sense of community offered by the mobile home park, by the stability of her mother's workplace, and even by the policies that brought her family back to the Lower Ninth Ward to become actively engaged in the community's redevelopment.

All of this leads to a central question: Is it possible to design policies, programs, and interventions to replicate such resilience? Is it feasible to identify the factors that promote such "resilient" outcomes among children and youth, either directly or indirectly, and then target interventions to enhance, activate, or facilitate these factors? Resilience is complex, operating at multiple intersecting levels that encompass individual biology, cognition, and psychology; family dynamics; communal and institutional support systems; and policy environments. This puzzle reflects a fundamental question that has been posed by Yehuda and colleagues (2006): "Are resilient people born, or made?"

INTRODUCTION

In this white paper, we consider the current science and practice of resilience interventions for children and youth[1] who are susceptible to disasters or who have been exposed to disasters. Starting from the central question introduced in the prologue above—is it possible to design evidence-based resilience interventions for children?—this paper reviews the ways in which resilience research has influenced resilience interventions, considers specific illustrations of these resilience practices, and examines the evidentiary base for these activities. Furthermore, we will place these disaster-related resilience interventions within a public health framework of primary, secondary, and tertiary prevention. Public

[1]In the interest of editorial brevity, throughout this white paper, we will mainly refer to children and youth, across the age spectrum of toddler to adolescent, as "children"

health may have entered the field of resilience interventions rather late in the game, but its community-based practice orientation and methods for assessing programmatic effectiveness and theoretical construct fidelity can offer powerful tools to this burgeoning field of "interventional resilience." Lastly, we will explore the inherent challenges of developing evidence-based resilience practices within the context of disasters.

The field of resilience research has evolved in the 50 years since developmental psychologists first began examining what factors contributed to the positive social, emotional, and intellectual growth of children growing up in the face of highly adverse conditions, such as being reared by a schizophrenic parent (Garmezy, 1985; Garmezy et al., 1984) or living in environments of extreme poverty (Masten, 2001). Researchers noted that deficit models that focused on correlations among a child's personality, environment, and subsequent psychopathology were inadequate frameworks for providing robust explanations of how children developed. The goal was not merely to avoid psychopathology in children, but also to understand how children achieved their cognitive, social, and emotional potential. By contrasting children who were more successful at reaching key developmental milestones despite their adverse circumstances with those who were less successful, effectively illuminating what made them resilient, researchers hypothesized that they could articulate adaptation mechanisms. After these adaptation pathways were understood, the subsequent step would involve developing interventions that stimulated or facilitated these growth processes to encourage better outcomes for more children, regardless of their circumstances.

As a number of scholars have noted, this field of "positive psychology" spawned a short list of factors that were persistently associated with children's ability to adapt and achieve developmental milestones despite being exposed to chronic and acute adverse conditions (Luthar and Cicchetti, 2000; Luthar et al., 2006; Masten, 2001, 2008; Masten and Obradovic, 2008; Wright et al., 2013). These factors included child-specific characteristics such as good cognitive abilities; positive constructs of self (including self-efficacy and self-control); attitudinal and belief systems that encompassed hopefulness, faith, and a positive worldview; and the ability to form and sustain relationships with parents, peers, and siblings. Studies of American soldiers who were held captive in Vietnamese prisoner-of-war camps for extended periods revealed many of the same characteristics of resilience among adults (Yehuda et al., 2006).

Scholars have long noted that children do not grow up in a vacuum, but are embedded in a number of concentric social systems that support and nourish them—notably, their parents, their households, their peers, the institutions with which they interact, their communities, and society as a whole (Bronfenbrenner, 1986)—all of which exert an influence on children's ability to adapt to adverse conditions. Factors across all of these domains are often divided into two categories: those that "promote" adaptive competencies in children, and those that "protect" them from the negative consequences of exposure to adverse events leading to psychopathologies or stunted development. Wright and colleagues (2013) have referred to this phase of inquiry in the scientific evolution as the first two of four waves of resilience research: the first wave identified resilience factors, and the second wave explored resilience processes within individuals and across these multiple social systems.

With each succeeding wave, the resilience research field expanded beyond the original boundaries of developmental psychology. Wright et al. (2013) referred to the third wave as the examination of interventions that might enhance or facilitate resilience, and the still-emerging fourth wave is focused on a consideration of multiple system effects, notably within the fields of epigenetics and neurobiology. In the second and third waves, social scientists, education researchers, and social epidemiologists applied their disciplinary perspectives, particularly as the research explored the intersection of multiple levels (e.g., How does one measure a family or community's social capital and its relationship to a child's ability to adapt?); the relationship of resilience to health outcomes (including the biological mechanisms of action of adverse events triggering stress responses, which, in turn, lead to biochemical and genetic changes); and the institutional settings most conducive to resilience interventions for children (e.g., schools and day care centers).

These succeeding waves of resilience research have resulted in significant analytical shifts in the field as well. What began in the first wave as qualitative case-based research and quantitative variable-based research that generally relied on correlational analyses such as regression modeling, analysis of covariance, and categorical data analyses has evolved to include hierarchical modeling; latent growth curve analyses (particularly when looking at the relationship of resilience factors compared to recovery over time) (Bonanno et al., 2011); structural equation and propensity score modeling (Abramson et al., 2010b, Stehling-Ariza et al., 2012); and complex system science approaches (Sherrieb et al., 2010). The benefit of such sophisticated analyses is that they permit far more nuanced tests of frameworks and models that can incorporate multiple social levels, as well as dimensions of time. The cost to such complexity is that it may be regarded as out of reach for a practice community eager to translate such findings in to programs and interventions.

As different scientific communities struggled with finding common ground in defining, operationalizing, and analyzing resilience, the concept of population resilience emerged in political discourse as well, particularly during the past decade. In 2005, the United Nations secretariat of the International Strategy for Disaster Reduction convened 168 countries in Japan, culminating in the Hyogo Framework for Action. This international blueprint for risk reduction urged countries to develop national resilience programs and strategies to reduce the impacts of natural disasters. In response, political leaders in a number of countries, including the United States and Canada, called for national resilience efforts. For example, the 2009 U.S. National Health Security Strategy has two goals, the first of which is to "build community resilience" and the second of which is to strengthen health and emergency response systems. This foundational policy document goes on to elaborate that

> Communities help build resilience by implementing policies and practices to ensure the conditions under which people can be healthy, by assuring access to medical care, building social cohesion, supporting healthy behaviors, and creating a culture of preparedness in which bystander response to emergencies is not the exception but the norm.

In Presidential Policy Directive 8, issued in 2011, resilience is defined as "the ability to *adapt* to changing conditions and *withstand* and *rapidly recover* from disruption due to emergencies" [emphasis added] (Brown, 2011).

This political rhetoric has translated to administrative action as well. Among the notable mandates are the Centers for Disease Control and Prevention's (CDC's) *Public Health Emergency Preparedness Capabilities: National Standards for State and Local Planning* (2011), which lists community preparedness and community recovery as the two capabilities that every public health department should plan for as part of their "community resilience" domain. State and public health agencies, in turn, are tasked with identifying processes and outcome measures that can demonstrate to their satisfaction, and that of their federal funders, that they are engaging in and achieving "community resilience." Although these appear to be entirely different constructs from individual resilience, as Norris and colleagues (2008) pointed out in their seminal article on community resilience, (a) the concept of resilience is often viewed metaphorically rather than operationally (in that it represents a return to a prior steady state after being shocked or deformed, and thus may be viewed as either an outcome or a dynamic process), and (b) community resilience is often measured as the capacity to sustain individual physical and mental health and well-being within a community

(Norris et al., 2008). The combination of the definitional ambiguity and the potential interpretation of community resilience as the aggregation of individually resilient residents suggests considerable measurement challenges.

In addition to scientific and governmental interest in cultivating "resilience interventions," there has been increasing awareness and attention to the specific risks associated with children who have been exposed to natural, technological, and manmade disasters (NCCD, 2010; Peek, 2008). Despite the apparent rarity of a disaster happening in any one individual's life, in recent years the number of domestic disasters and complex emergencies affecting children and youth has increased—including several high-profile events such as the World Trade Center attacks (Hoven et al., 2003); Hurricane Katrina (Abramson et al., 2008; McLaughlin et al., 2009); the BP oil spill (Abramson et al., 2010a); the Joplin, Missouri, tornado; the Newtown, Connecticut, school shooting; and, most recently, the Moore, Oklahoma, tornado. In addition to these major events, children are exposed to any number of "smaller" communal disasters, including flooding, wildfires, and mass traumas. The acute phases of a disaster inevitably lead to secondary stresses on children and youth: displacement, academic interruptions and disruptions, social network cleavages, and economic and mobility constraints. These initial and secondary stresses lead to many consequences, some of them invisible for years. Among these are physical health effects and increased rates of chronic health conditions that emerge across the lifespan; immediate and enduring mental health effects, including self-limiting posttraumatic stress disorder, behavioral and emotional disturbance, and complicated grief; educational disadvantages, including missed grade promotions; and social role effects. Alongside this increased awareness and understanding of the many complex effects of disasters on children has been a growing emphasis by governmental, philanthropic, and voluntary sectors on identifying and intervening to promote positive development among children and avert long-term morbidity and pathology.

Cumulatively, these various interests, the evolving science, and the pressing demands to address children's needs post-disaster have led to an increasing appreciation of the need to develop evidence-based resilience interventions.

THE LANDSCAPE OF DISASTER-RELATED RESILIENCE INTERVENTIONS FOR CHILDREN

We employed several search strategies to identify programs and interventions whose expressed goals and objectives were to enhance children's resiliency and to identify evidence of the effectiveness of resilience interventions. The initial Internet search for programs was conducted using the following search terms: "youth empowerment program," "youth leadership programs," "disaster preparedness [or] recovery," "youth [or] child resilience," and "disaster education." Based on these search criteria, a limited number of programs were identified. A second search was conducted in which we added identifiers for specific disasters: "Hurricane Katrina," "Hurricane Rita," "Joplin tornado," "April 2011 tornados," "2010 Midwest floods," "2010 Arkansas floods," "2007 California wildfires," and "9/11 terror attacks." Lastly, programs were further identified and researched as they arose throughout the literature search. For instance, programs referenced by articles uncovered during the literature search were included in the list of programs. Each program or intervention was reviewed to determine if it intentionally addressed any of the "short list" of resilience factors identified in the literature (Wright et al., 2013). A total of 17 programs were identified; these are listed in Tables G-1 and G-2. This is not intended to be an exhaustive list of all resilience programs or interventions, but rather an illustrative list.

As depicted in Table G-1, we have characterized resilience interventions according to moderating and mediating factors that correspond to the most commonly cited predictors of child resilience. The interventions may be intended directly for the children and youth or for the parents or household, or be targeted to larger social spheres such as child-oriented institutions or the community at large. For each mediating or moderating factor, we have further distinguished the programmatic objectives of the interventions. For example, there are resilience interventions that focus on promoting "self-identity," and within that domain there are distinct programmatic objectives of enhancing self-efficacy and others for enhancing self-esteem. We have also characterized each of the intervention's objectives by where it would fit in a public health prevention model. Given that these disaster resilience programs are often similar in size and scale to community-based health promotion and disease prevention programs, and that there may be advantages to aligning the resilience programs with similar programs that target risk reduction or skill enhancement among children and youth, we have categorized the interventions as fitting within primary, secondary, or tertiary prevention models:

- **Primary prevention programs** target populations who are potentially exposed to disaster, and their objective is to prevent exposure to, or consequences of, adverse or toxic agents. This is consistent with the definition of resilience as "withstanding" or resisting the disaster exposure. Much of the programmatic activity in these programs occurs before the disaster.
- **Secondary prevention programs** target populations who were exposed to disaster but for whom it is unknown whether or to what extent they were affected. The objective of these programs is to "treat" populations to minimize the debilitating effects of disaster exposure. This is consistent with the definition of resilience as "adapting," and generally occurs after the disaster and the exposure.
- **Tertiary prevention programs** target populations who were exposed *and* affected; their objective is to facilitate rapid and complete recovery and prevent "spread" to others or deterioration of the health of the population. This is consistent with the definition of resilience as "rapid recovery," and exclusively occurs after the disaster exposure.

Table G-2 describes the specific programs that illustrate the resilience objectives in Table G-1.

Overall, it is noteworthy how few programs were identified using these search criteria, and it suggests that the field of "interventional resilience" programming for children and youth is still evolving. It is likely that a number of programs have been developed in response to disasters, but are implemented locally with little documentation or evaluation of their effectiveness. Furthermore, we are aware of a number of programs in development whose express purpose is to enhance child and youth resilience through targeted interventions, but they are in the early stages of design and implementation. It is also important to note that we have purposefully excluded the many non-disaster resilience programs that exist (Head Start and 4-H programs, for example), because disaster context is often quite distinct from chronic adversities or more routine environments. We also elected to exclude programs or interventions that were narrowly focused on mental health treatment only, even in post-disaster settings.

Many of the programs and interventions we identified were built on preparedness education models, in which children and youth were taught the basics of emergency preparedness, given risk-specific instructions (such as seeking shelter in tornado-susceptible areas or bomb shelters in war zones), and taught specific survival and recovery skills. These interventions were often classroom-based (e.g., Minnesota's Disaster Readiness Actions for Teens, Wisconsin's READY program, American Red Cross' Masters of Disaster, Israel's Urban Resilience Program), but a number were also community-based (such as the Boy Scouts, Girl Scouts, or Teen Community Emergency Response Team [CERT]). Many of these programs are explicitly intended to enhance self-efficacy and provide opportunities for helping others, although we have attempted to characterize these programs by their presumed or implicit objectives, notwithstanding their stated programmatic goals. Virtually all of these education-based interventions occur in the pre-disaster stage and are generally intended to promote moderating traits among children and youth. In addition, they develop facets within youth that may be "mobilized" during a disaster and that can serve as risk-activated moderators.

Several of the programs and interventions promote very specific social and emotional skills, including stress-reduction techniques (e.g., Israel's Urban Resilience Program), communication and relationship-building techniques (e.g., Journey of Hope), or political advocacy skills (e.g., the Vietnamese American Young Leaders Association [VAYLA] and the Rethinkers, both in New Orleans). These skill-oriented programs are a combination of pre- and post-disaster activities and appear to be most effective as primary prevention models when they are tied to specific risks or hazards.

Three programs in particular—Save the Children's Resilient and Ready Community Initiatives, the Communities Advancing Resilience Toolkit, and the Joplin Child Care Task Force—focus on community-wide policies, infrastructure, governance and response entities, and child-oriented institutions rather than directly on the children or youth. Their objectives fit more properly into larger ecological models of resilience, in which children's well-being is contingent on the stability and competency of multiple institutions affecting their lives. We have included these broader community-oriented programs in the program matrix because they explicitly reference children's well-being and resilience as a programmatic objective.

A number of the resilience interventions seek to broaden children and youth's worldviews, offering historical, political, and social context to disaster events and their consequences. These include the New York City–based 9/12 project that emerged after the September 11 attacks, Israel's Urban Resilience Program, VAYLA and the Rethinkers programs in New Orleans, and FEMA's Youth Advisory Council. Although these programs differ in their perspectives, all offer youth explanatory frameworks for disaster risk and consequence that promote hopefulness and agency for the children. These programs are a mix of pre- and post-disaster interventions, and thus serve both primary and secondary prevention goals.

Across all these resilience interventions, however, there is very limited evaluation of their effectiveness or representation of a clear evidence base that reflects interventions mapped to theoretical constructs that had been measured and analyzed. Although the research literature offers substantial evidencc on the relationship of child, parental, and communal characteristics to child development, the evidence for programmatic effectiveness is extraordinarily shallow. The next section considers some of the challenges in developing such an evidence base for resilience interventions.

TABLE G-1 Child and Youth Resilience Interventions

Moderators/ Mediators	Objective	Prevention/Intervention		
		Primary	**Secondary**	**Tertiary**
Self-Identity	Increase self-efficacy	• Masters of Disaster* • Teen Community Emergency Response Team (CERT)* • Youth Preparedness Council • Emergency Preparedness Award, Boy Scouts • Emergency Preparedness Patch, Girl Scouts • STEP Program, READY camp and class • Disaster Readiness Actions for Teens (DRAT)*	• Vietnamese American Young Leaders Association (VAYLA)* • Rethinkers	
	Increase self-worth and self-esteem	• Youth Preparedness Council	• Rethinkers	
Self-Control	Increase executive control and self-regulation	• Urban Resilience Program* • DRAT*		
Coping Skill-Building	Increase problem-solving competence	• Youth Preparedness Council • Emergency Preparedness Award, Boy Scouts	• Rethinkers	

		• Masters of Disaster* • Emergency Preparedness Patch, Girl Scouts • Urban Resilience Program**		
	Teach stress reduction	• Urban Resilience Program*	• Child Friendly Spaces Program* • Urban Resilience Program** • Journey of Hope***	• Joplin Child Care Task Force
Relationship Enhancement	Improve parenting skills		• Resilient and Ready Communities Initiative* • Joplin Child Care Task Force	
	Improve family dynamics and communication	• Resilient and Ready Communities Initiative* • Communities Advancing Resilience Toolkit (CART)	• Resilient and Ready Communities Initiative*	
	Identify or connect to trusted adults		• Child Friendly Spaces Program* • Journey of Hope*** • Rethinkers* • VAYLA*	

			• Joplin Child Care Task Force	
Opportunities for Pro-Social Behavior	Provide opportunities to help others	• Youth Preparedness Council • Teen CERT • DRAT* • Emergency Preparedness Award, Boy Scouts • Emergency Preparedness Patch, Girl Scouts	• Rethinkers* • VAYLA	
Enhanced or Increased Resources	Increase access to *human capital*, such as better health, emotional well-being, job skills, youth empowerment and development	• Resilient and Ready Communities Initiative • Teen CERT** • Urban Resilience Program** • CART	• Child Friendly Spaces Program* • Journey of Hope*** • The 9/12 Generation Project • Liberty's Kitchen • Rethinkers* • VAYLA*	• CHF Mobile Mental Health
	Increase access to *social capital*, including increased communication and social support	• Resilient and Ready Communities Initiative • Youth Preparedness Council • DRAT*	• Child Friendly Spaces Program* • Journey of Hope*** • Rethinkers* • VAYLA*	

	Increase access to *political capital*, such as the ability to advocate for oneself, one's community, and others	• Teen CERT* • Youth Preparedness Council • Rethinkers* • VAYLA*	• Rethinkers* • VAYLA*	
	Increase access to *economic capital*, such as resources, materials, and basic needs (clothing, etc.)		• Rethinkers* • VAYLA*	
Positive Worldview	Increase or develop communal solidarity	• Youth Preparedness Council • Urban Resilience Program** • DRAT* • The 9/12 Generation Project • Rethinkers* • VAYLA*	• Rethinkers* • VAYLA* • The 9/12 Generation Project	
	Contextualize and situate understanding of hazard or traumatic event so that attribution of cause is external rather than internal (effort to counter learned helplessness)		• Urban Resilience Program** • Rethinkers* • VAYLA* • The 9/12 Generation Project	• Rethinkers* • VAYLA*

Institutional Stability	Increase stability and support of schools, youth sports and programs, and day care, as well as primary and specialty care	• Resilient and Ready Communities Initiative • The 9/12 Generation Project	• Resilient and Ready Communities Initiative • Child Friendly Spaces Program*** • Journey of Hope*** • Rethinkers* • VAYLA* • Joplin Child Care Task Force
Resumption of Social Routines	Provide environment for or facilitate return to pre-disaster routines	• Urban Resilience Program** • The 9/12 Generation Project	• Child Friendly Spaces Program*** • Journey of Hope***
Social Order/Stability	Address community-wide issues of social disruptions, inequality, and stability of social institutions such as schools, health care facilities, and criminal justice systems		• Rethinkers* • VAYLA*

*Process or program evaluation (accomplishes program objectives).
**Intermediate impact (intervention achieved intermediate objectives).
***Outcome impact (intervention either promotes recovery, decreases pathology, increases educational attainment/objective).

TABLE G-2 Youth-Oriented Program Descriptions

Program	Target Audience	Setting	Objectives
9/12 Generation Project (New York Says Thank You Foundation)	Youth, middle, and high school students	Community	Activate students in service-learning projects focused on community revitalization, disaster relief, and the arts; empower students to engage in positive impacts beyond their immediate communities and economic means; encourage solidarity among students and youth nationwide; provide positive lessons arising from disaster
Child Friendly Spaces Program (Save the Children)	Children, youth, caregivers, disaster-affected communities	Post-disaster, shelters, places of congregation post-emergency	Provide stable space for children to play, socialize, and begin to recover post-disaster with the goal of protecting children from harm and providing a sense of normalcy and community; educate leaders to meet needs of children
Communities Advancing Resilience Toolkit (Terrorism and Disaster Center of the National Child Traumatic Stress Network)	Communities	Community	Community intervention process for community action planning; encourage community relationships and resilience, prompt community members to assess needs, generate community profiles, develop strategic plans, and implement these plans
Disaster Readiness Actions for Teens (Minnesota	Youth	Community	Provide emergency preparedness training for teens by engaging, educating, and empowering youth to respond safely during critical incidents; utilizes a "train-the-trainer" concept to educate teens to come together to teach others about preparedness

Department of Health)			
Emergency Preparedness Award (Boy Scouts of America)	Youth, boys	Community	Educate and empower young men to respond when disaster strikes; provide opportunity to help others during emergency
Emergency Preparedness Patch (Girl Scouts Council of the Nation's Capital)	Youth, girls	Community	Motivate and empower young women to become leaders in emergency management and response; provide opportunity to help others during emergency
Joplin Child Care Task Force	Youth	Community	Community-based collaboration to respond to children's and providers' mental health needs; provide stable space for children to play, socialize, and begin to recover post-disaster with the goal of protecting children from harm and providing a sense of normalcy and community; educate leaders to meet needs of children
Journey of Hope (Save the Children)	Youth	Community	Provide caregivers and youth with the support, education, training, and resources necessary to understand and normalize emotions associated with hardships; support children and caregivers in developing positive coping strategies to deal with their emotions; build on the inner strengths of children, families, schools, and communities to further develop positive coping strategies; develop a person's sense of hope and future by empowering him or her to feel more in control
Masters of Disaster (American Red Cross)	Youth	School, community	Ready-to-go kit designed to integrate lessons of disaster into regular school lesson plans; provide disaster safety instruction to students and families; help students and families understand and prepare for disasters; educate youth on how to stay safe and help others during and after a disaster
Mobile Medical and Community	Youth	Community, school	Provide primary medical and mental health care to children in individual settings and provide group activities to facilitate communication; utilize

Resilience Support Units (Children's Health Fund)			"coping boxes" and play therapy with younger children; promote healthy development and emotional well-being
Resilient and Ready Communities Initiative	Youth, children, caregivers, communities	Community	Community-based approach to help local communities address the needs of children in disasters; reduce impact of disasters and emergencies on children through effective preparedness, response, recovery, and advocacy; help at-risk regions meet national standards and integrate best practices to support children's safety and well-being through preparedness planning and programs
Rethinkers (New Orleans public schools)	Youth	New Orleans public schools	Empower youth to identify needs in their post-disaster community and advocate effectively for reform; provide youth with the skills necessary to take action to improve their educational experience
STEP Program, READY Camp and Class (Wisconsin Center for School, Youth, and Citizen Preparedness)	Youth, teachers	Community, school (Wisconsin)	Educate and prepare youth and teachers to respond and recover from serious, unexpected situations; empower youth to take control of their safety by developing emergency plans for themselves and their families; train youth to help themselves and others during emergencies
Teen Community Emergency Response Training (CERT) (Federal Emergency Management Agency)	Youth	Community, school	Educate youth about disaster preparedness for hazards specific to their community to ensure they have the skills needed to protect themselves and assist others; prepare and address response capabilities in high schools; train students in school security and emergency response procedures; involve youth in the country's overall emergency preparedness and basic response plans

Urban Resilience Program (Cohen-Harris Center)	Youth	School (Israel)	Prepare youth and the population to cope with the consequences of disasters and reinforce citizen resilience; aid communities in developing function, social flexibility, and a means of coping through community capital, resilience and education
Vietnamese American Young Leaders Association of New Orleans	Youth	Community (New Orleans)	Promote youth development and community empowerment through cultural awareness, education, and engagement; empower youth through supportive services and organizing for cultural enrichment and positive social change
Youth Preparedness Council	Youth	National	Promote youth empowerment, preparedness, and resiliency through the experience of peer discussion and learning; educate and promote youth to serve on a national council and bring their experiences back to their communities to help develop and advance local preparedness and resilience

EVALUATING THE EVIDENCE BASE FOR RESILIENCE INTERVENTIONS

At a minimum, there appear to be at least three types of challenges to the development of an evidence base for resilience interventions: definitional, operational, and political. These are above and beyond the simpler explanation that this is still a young field, particularly in the context of disasters, and that it will take time for the programs to be sufficiently developed to allow for robust evaluations and accumulation of evidence.

- **Definitional challenges:**
  - Resilience outcomes are not universal or standardized. Even distinguishing between the ability to withstand, adapt, or recover quickly reflects vastly different outcomes, and there is still a vigorous debate about whether resilience is a process, a latent construct, or a specific outcome. Furthermore, resilience can only be measured in the presence of (or in response to) an adverse or potentially traumatic event, thus complicating pre-disaster baseline measurement.
  - There is still considerable debate about whether resilience is defined as the absence of mental health pathology, the achievement of a specific developmental milestone, or the representation of a specific constellation of positive attributes (e.g., self-efficacy, positive worldview, etc.). The latter also raises the question of whether resilience may be subjectively or objectively measured.
  - Because of the recent interest in resilience across many disciplines and sectors, there are numerous methodologies and disciplinary lexicons that do not necessarily align.
- **Operational challenges:**
  - The processes and factors underlying resilience are extraordinarily complex, operating at multiple levels that include biological, psychological, social, and cultural domains. Analytical techniques such as systems science and structural equation modeling are being employed to handle these complex designs, although the value of such approaches will require many replicated studies. The statistical complexity also limits its accessibility to researchers and stakeholders. Beyond that, the multidisciplinary nature of these complex research questions and designs requires scientists and scholars who can understand and apply theory and methods from areas of expertise far beyond their own.

- The nature of much resilience research is that it relies on observational data, which is daunting for a number of reasons. The events themselves are rare and unpredictable; it is difficult to get into the field quickly enough to collect critical time-series data; there are rarely accessible pre-disaster data available; and it is particularly difficult to control for competing explanations in such quasi-experimental research.
- It has also been difficult to operationalize the effects of formal help mechanisms in observational studies because they are so varied, are not universally defined, and have no common data systems. The problems inherent in such resilience research are common to public health research's efforts to evaluate community health interventions, and solutions in that field may find traction in resilience research.
- Exposure itself may be related to social vulnerability factors, which limit researchers' ability to develop case-control strategies contingent on exposure.

- **Political challenges:**
  - Domestically, the federal government does not generally provide or fund disaster-related child resilience services, strategies, or programs, and therefore has little institutional interest in funding evaluation research (Abramson et al., 2007; Garrett et al., 2007).
  - Most of the extant programming has emerged from the nonprofit, philanthropic, and humanitarian aid sectors, which have limited funding for rigorous evaluation methods, and which favor programmatic dollars over research dollars.
  - "Root-cause" theories and frameworks suggest the need for interventions that are (a) complex, (b) socially progressive, (c) structural, and (d) not the responsibility of any one sector or domain (meaning that there is little accountability or demand for an evidentiary base). As such, there is a limited political advocacy coalition that can advocate for federal research funding, particularly in times of constrained and shrinking science budgets.

MOVING FORWARD WITH "INTERVENTIONAL RESILIENCE"

Despite the challenges noted above, there are several noteworthy trends or opportunities in resilience research. The first is the notion of expanding existing youth programs that have the capacity to "reach forward" into disaster settings. The Boy Scouts and Girl Scouts are examples of such programs, but it is easy to imagine that other well-established youth-empowerment and youth-development programs (such as 4-H) could be expanded in to disaster realms. This would provide control groups of children who have not been exposed to disaster. Just as there is possibility for reaching forward, there is evidence of "reaching back," when disaster-inspired programs, such as VAYLA and Rethinkers, establish themselves in communities as progressive (but non-disaster) youth-empowerment programs. This extends the utility of such programs and also affords the research community the ability to test the effect of disaster context on resilience outcomes (as do the reaching-forward programs).

As mentioned earlier in this white paper, there are also public health research strategies that can be employed in resilience research. There is a long history in public health of community-based research; the Healthy Communities movement, social medicine, and social determinants of health models align both theoretically and programmatically with a number of resilience interventions. There are well-developed evaluation and meta-review strategies, such as the Cochrane Collaborative and CDC's *Community Preventive Services Guide*, which can serve as models for programmatic evaluations. The field of social epidemiology in particular has embraced complex systems sciences, which can be applied to many multilevel resilience research strategies.

This brings us back to "M," the hardy Katrina survivor and her daughter who were profiled briefly in the prologue. In thinking about bottling the resilience factors in their lives and designing interventions that can be applied to others, a number of possibilities emerge. First, to the extent possible, create programs and policies that allow children to remain within their educational environments, assuming that these were positive and high-quality environments. Develop family-based programs that bring parents and children together to create and employ coping skills (like the scrapbook "M" created) that can further enhance familial closeness and communication. Create community-focused emergency housing environments for populations that may be displaced for long periods of time to allow for collective self-efficacy and communal solidarity. Finally, develop programs that empower children and families to be actively involved in rebuilding their own communities, as a means of affirming their self-efficacy and countering the social role of "victim."

That said, we do not know with any certainty that these strategies are effective or, rather, which parts of these strategies exert what effect, and to what end? Of course, in the absence of hard evidence, we can certainly follow the five principles offered by Hobfoll and colleagues (2007) in the design of *any* resilience intervention: (1) promote safety, (2) promote calming, (3) promote self- and collective efficacy, (4) promote connectedness, and (5) instill hope.

REFERENCES

Abramson, D. M., S. S. Morse, A. L. Garrett, and I. Redlener. 2007. Public health disaster research: Surveying the field, defining its future. *Disaster Medicine and Public Health Preparedness* 1(1):57-62.

Abramson, D., T. Stehling-Ariza, R. Garfield, and I. Redlener. 2008. Prevalence and predictors of mental health distress post-Katrina: Findings from the Gulf Coast Child and Family Health Study. *Disaster Medicine and Public Health Preparedness* 2(2):77-86.

Abramson, D., I. Redlener, T. Stehling-Ariza, J. Sury, A. Banister, and Y. S. Park. 2010a. *Impact on Children and Families of the Deepwater Horizon Oil Spill: Preliminary Findings of the Coastal Population Impact Study*. New York: National Center for Disaster Preparedness, Columbia University.

Abramson, D. M., T. Stehling-Ariza, Y. S. Park, L. Walsh, and D. Culp. 2010b. Measuring individual disaster recovery: A socioecological framework. *Disaster Medicine and Public Health Preparedness* 4(Suppl 1):S46-S54.

Bonanno, G. A., M. Westphal, and A. D. Mancini. 2011. Resilience to loss and potential trauma. *Annual Review of Clinical Psychology* 7:511-535.

Bronfenbrenner, U. 1986. Ecology of the family as a context for human development: Research perspectives. *Developmental Psychology* 22(6):723-742.

Brown, J. T. 2011. *Presidential Policy Directive 8 and the National Preparedness System: Background and Issues for Congress*. Washington, DC: Congressional Research Service, R42073.

CDC (Centers for Disease Control and Prevention). 2011. *Public Health Preparedness Capababilities: National Standards for State and Local Planning*. http://www.cdc.gov/phpr/capabilities/Capabilities_March_2011.pdf (accessed April 4, 2011).

Garmezy, N. 1985. Stress resistant children: The search for protective factors. In *Recent Research in Developmental Psychology, Journal of Child Psychology and Psychiatry* (Book Supplement No. 4). Oxford: Pergamon Press. Pp. 213-233.

Garmezy, N., A. S. Masten, and A. Tellegen. 1984. The study of stress and competence in children: A building block for developmental psychopathology. *Child Development* 55(1):97-111.

Garrett, A. L., R. Grant, P. Madrid, A. Brito, D. Abramson, and I. Redlener. 2007. Children and megadisasters: Lessons learned in the new millennium. *Advances in Pediatrics* 54:189-214.

Hobfoll, S., P. J. Watson, C. W. Bell, R. A. Bryant, M. J. Brymer, M. J. Friedman, M. Friedman, B. P. R. Gersons, J. T. V. M. de Jong, C. M. Layne, S. Maguen, Y. Neria, A. E. Norwood, R. Pynoos, D. Reissman, J. I. Ruzek, A. Y. Shalev, Z. Solomon, A. M. Steinberg, and R. J. Ursano. 2007. Five essential elements of immediate and mid-term mass trauma intervention: Empirical evidence. *Psychiatry* 70(4):283-315.

Hoven, C. W., C. S. Duarte, and D. J. Mandell. 2003. Children's mental health after disasters: The impact of the World Trade Center attack. *Current Psychiatry Reports* 5(2):101-107.

Luthar, S., and D. Cicchetti. 2000. The construct of resilience: Implications for interventions and social policies. *Development and Psychopathology* 12(04):857-885.

Luthar, S., D. J. Cohen, and D. Cicchetti. 2006. Resilience in development: A synthesis of research across five decades. *Developmental Psychopathology* 3.

Masten, A. S. 2001. Ordinary magic: Resilience processes in development. *American Psychologist* 56(3):227-238.

Masten, A. S. 2008. Resilience in developing systems: Progress and promise as the fourth wave rises. *Developmental Psychopathology* 19(3):921-930.

Masten, A. S., and J. Obradovic. 2008. Disaster preparation and recovery: Lessons from research on resilience in human development. *Ecology and Society* 13(1).

McLaughlin, K., J. A. Fairbank, M. J. Gruber, R. T. Jones, M. D. Lakoma, B. Pfefferbaum, N. A. Sampson, and R. C. Kessler. 2009. Serious emotional disturbance among youths exposed to Hurricane Katrina 2 years postdisaster. *Journal of the American Academy of Child and Adolescent Psychiatry* 48(11):1069-1078.

NCCD (National Commission on Children and Disasters). 2010. *2010 Report to the President and Congress*. Rockville, MD: Agency for Healthcare Research and Quality.

Norris, F., S. Stevens, B. Pfefferbaum, K. Wyche, and R. Pfefferbaum. 2008. Community resilience as a metaphor, theory, set of capacities, and strategy for disaster readiness. *American Journal of Community Psychology* 41(1):127-150.

Peek, L. 2008. Children and disasters: Understanding vulnerability, developing capacities, and promoting resilience—an introduction. *Children, Youth and Environments* 18(1):1-29.

Sherrieb, K., F. Norris, and S. Galea. 2010. Measuring capacities for community resilience. *Social Indicators Research* 99(2):227-247.

Stehling-Ariza, T., Y. S. Park, J. J. Sury, and D. Abramson. 2012. Measuring the impact of Hurricane Katrina on access to a personal healthcare provider: The use of the National Survey of Children's Health for an external comparison group. *Maternal and Child Health Journal* 16(Suppl 1):S170-S177.

Wright, M. O. D., A. S. Masten, and A. J. Narayan. 2013. Resilience processes in development: Four waves of research on positive adaptation in the context of adversity. In *Handbook of Resilience in Children*, edited by R. B. Brooks, and S. Goldstein. New York: Spinger Science Business Media. Pp. 15-37.

Yehuda, R., J. D. Flory, S. Southwick, and D. Charney. 2006. Developing an agenda for translational studies of resilience and vulnerability following trauma exposure. *Annals of the New York Academy of Sciences* 1071.

H

Recommendations from the National Commission on Children and Disasters

1. Disaster Management and Recovery

- Recommendation 1.1: Distinguish and comprehensively integrate the needs of children across all inter- and intra-governmental disaster management activities and operations.
- Recommendation 1.2: The President should accelerate the development and implementation of the National Disaster Recovery Framework with an explicit emphasis on addressing the immediate and long-term physical and mental health, educational, housing, and human services recovery needs of children.
- Recommendation 1.3: The Department of Homeland Security (DHS)/Federal Emergency Management Agency (FEMA) should ensure that information required for timely and effective delivery of recovery services to children and families is collected and shared with appropriate entities.
- Recommendation 1.4: DHS/FEMA should establish interagency agreements to provide disaster preparedness funding, technical assistance, training, and other resources to state and local child serving systems and child congregate care facilities.

2. Mental Health

- Recommendation 2.1: The Department of Health and Human Services (HHS) should lead efforts to integrate mental and behavioral health for children into public health, medical, and other relevant disaster management activities.

- Recommendation 2.2: HHS should enhance the research agenda for children's disaster mental and behavioral health, including psychological first aid, cognitive-behavioral interventions, social support interventions, bereavement counseling and support, and programs intended to enhance children's resilience in the aftermath of a disaster.
- Recommendation 2.3: Federal agencies and nonfederal partners should enhance pre-disaster preparedness and just-in-time training in pediatric disaster mental and behavioral health, including psychological first aid, bereavement support, and brief supportive interventions, for mental health professionals and individuals, such as teachers, who work with children.
- Recommendation 2.4: DHS/FEMA and the Substance Abuse and Mental Health Services Administration (SAMHSA) should strengthen the Crisis Counseling Assistance and Training Program (CCP) to better meet the mental health needs of children and families.
- Recommendation 2.5: Congress should establish a single, flexible grant funding mechanism to specifically support the delivery of mental health treatment services that address the full spectrum of behavioral health needs of children, including treatment of disaster-related adjustment difficulties, psychiatric disorders, and substance abuse.

3. Child Physical Health and Trauma

- Recommendation 3.1: Congress, HHS, and DHS/FEMA should ensure availability of and access to pediatric medical countermeasures (MCMs) at the federal, state, and local levels for chemical, biological, radiological, nuclear, and explosive threats.
- Recommendation 3.2: HHS and the Department of Defense (DoD) should enhance the pediatric capabilities of their disaster medical response teams through the integration of pediatric-specific training, guidance, exercises, supplies, and personnel.
- Recommendation 3.3: HHS should ensure that health professionals who may treat children during a disaster have adequate pediatric disaster clinical training.
- Recommendation 3.4: The Executive Branch and Congress should provide resources for a formal regionalized pediatric

system of care to support pediatric surge capacity during and after disasters.

- Recommendation 3.5: Prioritize the recovery of pediatric health and mental health care delivery systems in disaster-affected areas.
- Recommendation 3.6: The Environmental Protection Agency (EPA) should engage state and local health officials and non-governmental experts to develop and promote national guidance and best practices on re-occupancy of homes, schools, child care, and other child congregate care facilities in disaster-impacted areas.

4. Emergency Medical Services and Pediatric Transport

- Recommendation 4.1: The President and Congress should clearly designate and appropriately resource a lead federal agency for emergency medical services (EMS) with primary responsibility for the coordination of grant programs, research, policy, and standards development and implementation.
- Recommendation 4.2: Improve the capability of EMS to transport pediatric patients and provide comprehensive pre-hospital pediatric care during daily operations and disasters.
- Recommendation 4.3: HHS should develop a national strategy to improve federal pediatric emergency transport and patient care capabilities for disasters.

5. Disaster Case Management

- Recommendation 5.1: Disaster case management programs should be appropriately resourced and should provide consistent holistic services that achieve tangible, positive outcomes for children and families affected by the disaster.

6. Child Care and Early Education

- Recommendation 6.1: Congress and HHS should improve disaster preparedness capabilities for child care.
- Recommendation 6.2: Congress and federal agencies should improve capacity to provide child care services in the immediate aftermath of and recovery from a disaster.

- Recommendation 6.3: HHS should require disaster preparedness capabilities for Head Start Centers and basic disaster mental health training for staff.

7. Elementary and Secondary Education

- Recommendation 7.1: Congress and federal agencies should improve the preparedness of schools and school districts by providing additional support to states.
- Recommendation 7.2: Congress and the Department of Education should enhance the ability of school personnel to support children who are traumatized, grieving, or otherwise recovering from a disaster.
- Recommendation 7.3: Ensure that school systems recovering from disasters are provided immediate resources to reopen and restore the learning environment in a timely manner and provide support for displaced students and their host schools.

8. Child Welfare and Juvenile Justice

- Recommendation 8.1: Ensure that state and local child welfare agencies adequately prepare for disasters.
- Recommendation 8.2: Ensure that state and local juvenile justice agencies and all residential treatment, correctional, and detention facilities that house children adequately prepare for disasters.
- Recommendation 8.3: HHS and the Department of Justice (DOJ) should ensure that juvenile, dependency, and other courts hearing matters involving children adequately prepare for disasters.

9. Sheltering Standards, Services, and Supplies

- Recommendation 9.1: Government agencies and non-governmental organizations should provide a safe and secure mass care shelter environment for children, including access to essential services and supplies.

10. Housing

- Recommendation 10.1: Prioritize the needs of families with children, especially families with children who have disabilities or chronic health, mental health, or educational needs, within disaster housing assistance programs.

11. Evacuation

- Recommendation 11.1: Congress and federal agencies should provide sufficient funding to develop and deploy a national information sharing capability to quickly and effectively reunite displaced children with their families, guardians, and caregivers when separated by a disaster.
- Recommendation 11.2: Disaster plans at all levels of government must specifically address the evacuation and transportation needs of children with disabilities and chronic health needs, in coordination with child congregate care facilities such as schools, child care, and health care facilities.

SOURCE: National Commission on Children and Disasters. 2010. *Report to the President and Congress*. AHRQ Publication No. 10-M037, October 2010. Rockville, MD: Agency for Healthcare Research and Quality. http://www.ahrq.gov/prep/nccdreport (accessed September 8, 2013).